The Complete Low Fodmap Diet For Beginners

A Comprehensive Step-by-step Guide And Meal Plan To Manage IBS & Other Digestive Disorders

AMADAH HEATH

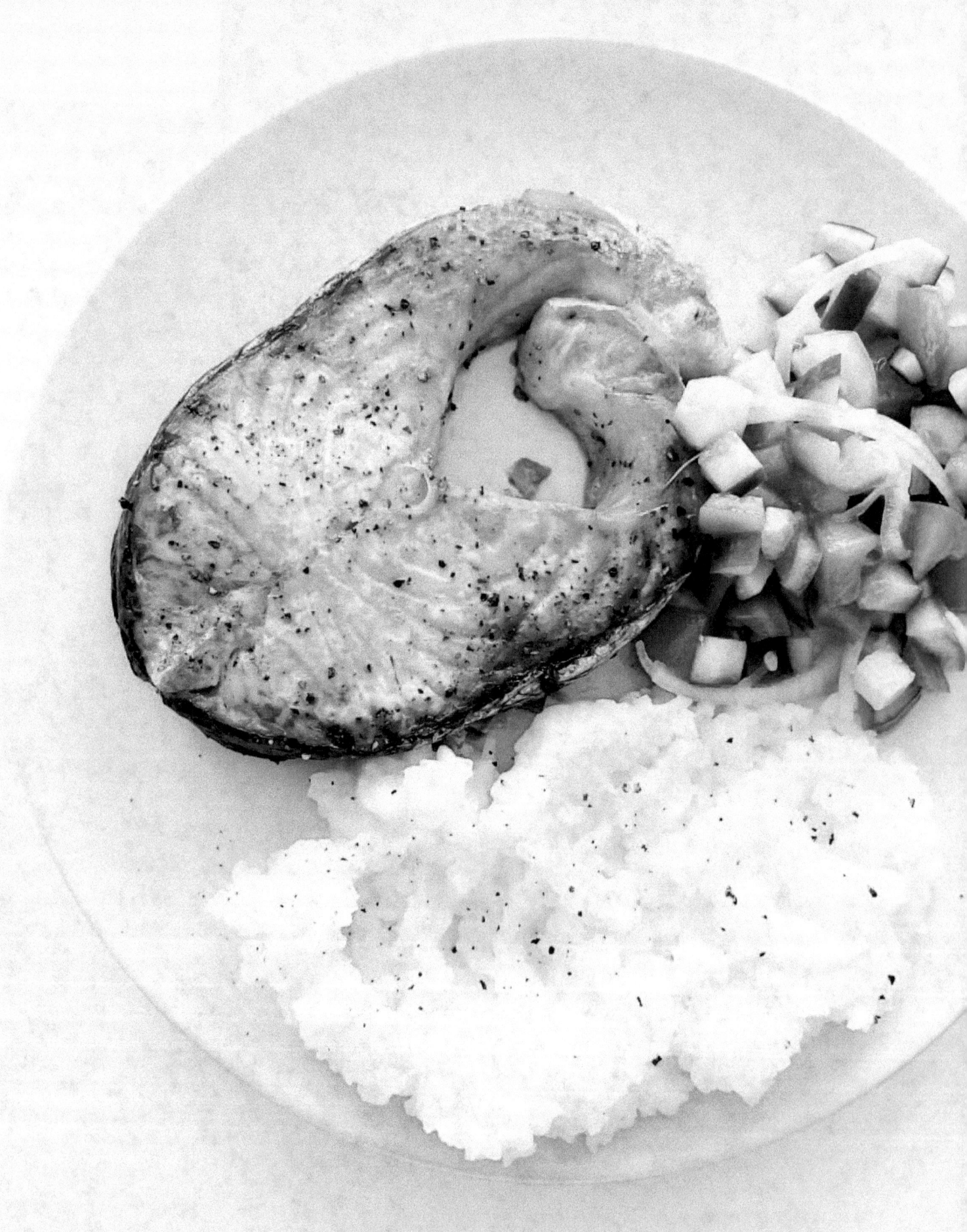

copyright

All rights reserved. No part of this book may be reproduced in any form or by any electronic or mechanical means, including information storage and retrieval systems, without permission in writing from the publisher, except by a reviewer, who may quote brief passages in a review.

Copyright © 2024 by Amada L. Heath

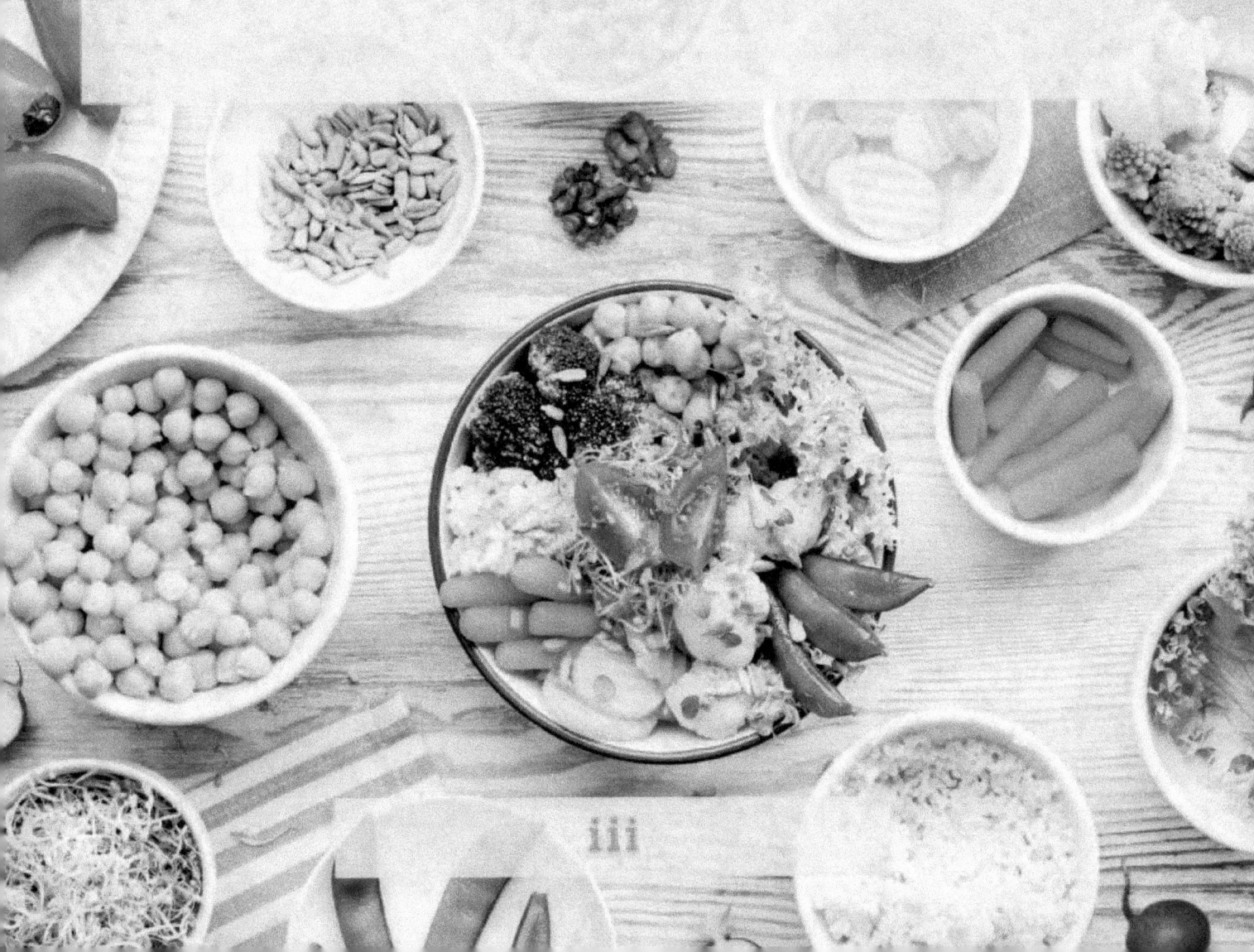

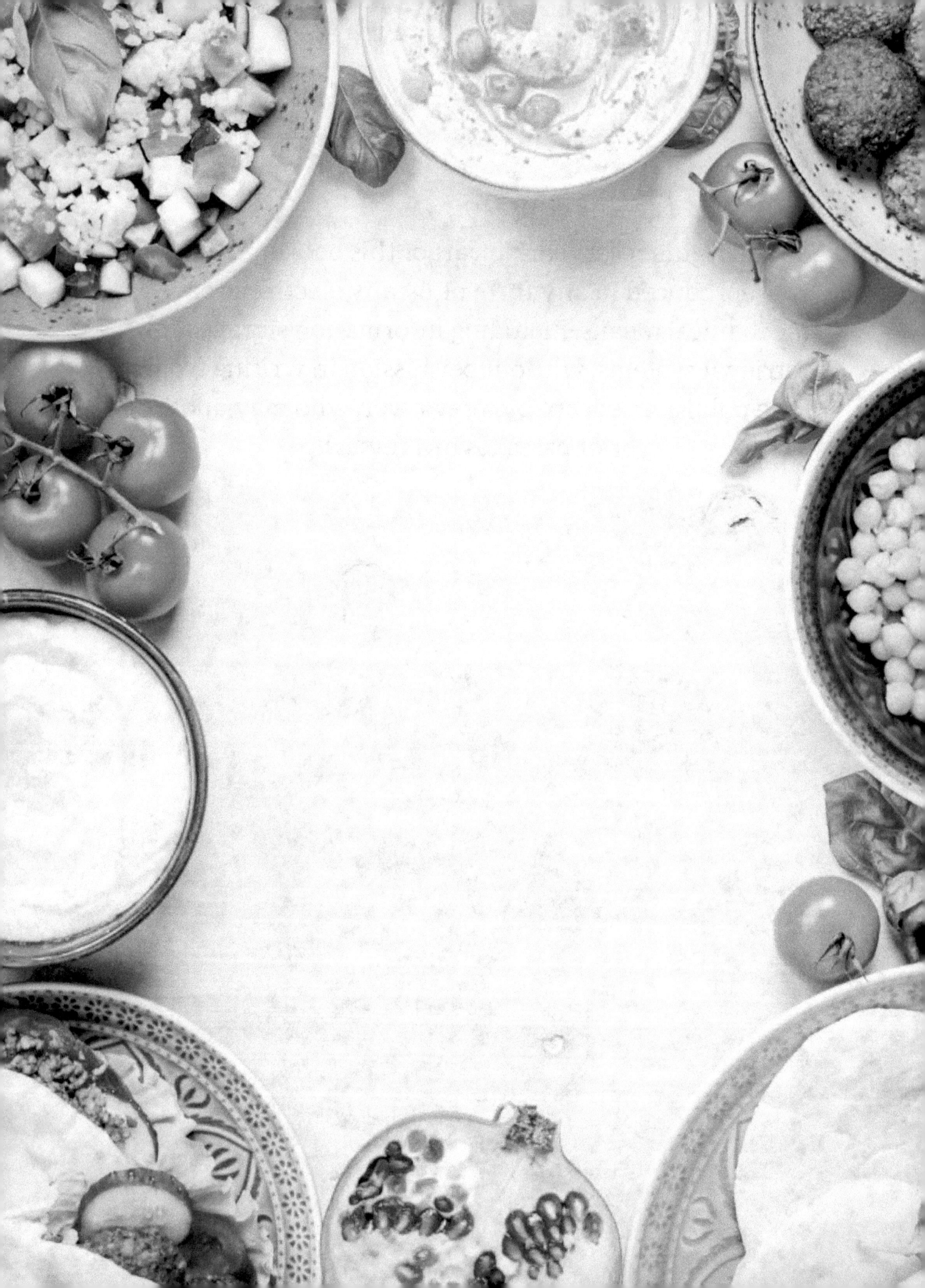

Table Of Contents

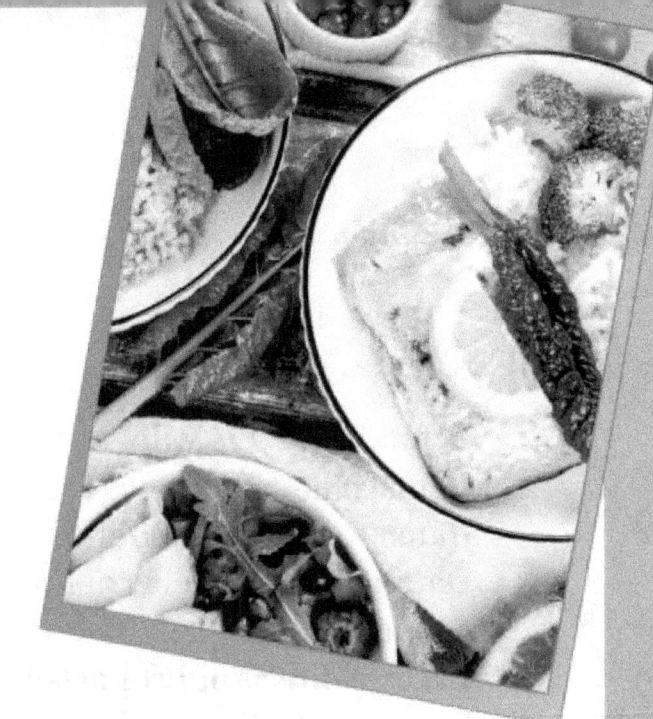

Introduction

How To Use This Book

Chapter 1

- Understanding the Low FODMAP Diet
- Role of FODMAPs in Gut Health
- Basics of the Low FODMAP Diet
- The Science Behind It: Phases Of The Low Fodmap Diet

Chapter 2

- Implementing The Low Fodmap Diet
- Benefits and Goals

Chapter 3

- Putting The Low Fodmap Diet Into Practice
- Low Fodmap Lifestyle and Digestive Health Tips

Chapter 4

- Cooking Tips And Modification

Healthy Friendly Recipes

Breakfast

- Scrambled Eggs with Spinach and Tomatoes
- Banana Almond Smoothie
- Oatmeal with Blueberries and Cinnamon
- Lactose-Free Yogurt Parfait
- Spinach and Cheese Omelet
- Peanut Butter Rice Cakes
- Quinoa Breakfast Bowl
- Coconut Chia Pudding
- Tomato and Basil Frittata
- Pumpkin Spice Overnight Oats
- Avocado Toast with Poached Egg
- Fruit and Cottage Cheese Bowl
- Almond Flour Pancakes
- Quinoa Breakfast Porridge
- Egg and Bell Pepper Cups
- Buckwheat Porridge with Strawberries
- Berry Chia Pudding
- Spinach and Feta Breakfast Wrap
- Maple-Cinnamon Rice Porridge
- Tomato & Basil Breakfast Skillet

Fish And Seafood

- Garlic-Infused Shrimp Stir-Fry
- Baked Cod with Dill and Lemon
- Pan-Seared Scallops with Lime
- Cilantro Lime Shrimp Skewers
- Sesame-Crusted Tuna Steaks
- Baked Tilapia with Paprika and Lemon
- Garlic-Infused Mackerel with Herbs
- Lemon-Ginger Baked Trout
- Herb-Crusted Baked Haddock
- Basil Lemon Grilled Swordfish
- Crispy Baked Sole Fillets
- Ginger Soy Shrimp Sauté
- Lemon Dill Poached Haddock
- Baked Mahi-Mahi with Fresh Herbs
- Paprika Grilled Prawns
- Sesame-Crusted Salmon
- Lime and Cilantro Grilled Tilapia
- Herb-Roasted Sea Bass
- Cumin-Spiced Grilled Halibut
- Chili Lime Grilled Tuna

Poultry

- Lemon Herb Grilled Chicken Breast
- Rosemary Baked Chicken Thighs
- Garlic-Infused Chicken Stir-Fry
- Basil Lime Chicken Skewers
- Paprika Baked Turkey Breast
- Ginger Lime Turkey Meatballs
- Balsamic Glazed Chicken Drumsticks
- Turmeric Lemon Roasted Chicken Wings
- Grilled Jerk-Spiced Chicken Thighs
- Cumin Spiced Grilled Turkey Breast
- Maple Mustard Chicken Breasts
- Citrus Grilled Chicken Thighs
- Rosemary Lemon Turkey Burgers
- Thyme Roasted Chicken Drumsticks
- Basil Pesto Baked Chicken
- Honey Lime Grilled Turkey Cutlets
- Sage Baked Chicken Breasts
- Teriyaki Turkey Stir-Fry
- Oregano Lemon Chicken Thighs
- Cumin Lime Grilled Chicken
- Cilantro Lime Turkey Meatballs

Vegetable And Salad

- Roasted Carrot and Zucchini Salad
- Spinach and Strawberry Salad
- Cucumber Dill Salad
- Roasted Bell Peppers and Eggplant
- Simple Tomato and Basil Salad
- Roasted Green Beans with Lemon Zest
- Grilled Asparagus with Sea Salt
- Carrot and Parsnip Mash
- Mixed Greens with Lemon Vinaigrette
- Roasted Butternut Squash with Thyme
- Roasted Sweet Potato and Spinach Salad
- Steamed Broccoli with Lemon Olive Oil
- Cabbage and Carrot Slaw
- Zucchini Noodles with Cherry Tomatoes
- Roasted Pumpkin with Rosemary
- Green Bean and Almond Salad
- Sautéed Kale with Lemon
- Carrot and Cucumber Ribbons Salad
- Grilled Bell Pepper Salad
- Roasted Fennel with Thyme
- Arugula and Lemon Salad

Snacks And Dessert

- Chocolate-Dipped Strawberries
- Cinnamon Almonds
- Peanut Butter Banana Bites
- Coconut Macaroons
- Baked Apple Slices
- Blueberry Yogurt Parfait
- Rice Cake with Avocado and Sea Salt
- Carrot Sticks with Hummus
- Kiwi and Coconut Popsicles
- Orange Dark Chocolate Bark
- Baked Banana Chips
- Coconut Chia Pudding
- Lactose-Free Yogurt with Kiwi and Walnuts
- Baked Cinnamon Apple Chips
- Chocolate Avocado Mousse
- Mixed Berry Smoothie
- Rice Cake with Peanut Butter and Blueberries
- Frozen Grape Snack
- Almond Butter Apple Slices
- Lemon Blueberry Muffins (Gluten-Free)

60-DAY MEAL PLAN

LIST OF INGREDIENTS

CONCLUSION

WEEKLY MEAL PLANNER

INTRODUCTION

Welcome to The Complete Low FODMAP Diet for Beginners, a comprehensive guide designed to help you navigate the world of Low FODMAP living with ease. If you're dealing with digestive issues like IBS (Irritable Bowel Syndrome) or other gastrointestinal discomforts, the Low FODMAP diet offers a scientifically-backed solution to managing and alleviating symptoms. If you've been struggling with constant bloating, painful cramps, unpredictable bowel movements, and an uneasy gut that seems to have a mind of its own, you're not alone. Digestive discomfort can overshadow your entire day, leaving you to worry about every meal and how it will affect your body. For those living with IBS or similar digestive disorders, this cycle is frustrating, exhausting, and can often feel like a battle you just can't win.

Maybe you've tried countless diets, medications, and "gut-friendly" foods, only to find yourself back at square one, enduring discomfort and distress. The uncertainty of not knowing which foods will trigger symptoms and disrupt your life can be mentally draining. Imagine never fully enjoying a meal with friends, hesitating to plan your day due to fear of flare-ups, or feeling anxious over what should be a nourishing experience. You deserve to eat without fear, to enjoy food again, and to have your life back.

This is where the Low FODMAP diet comes in—a scientifically proven approach to help you pinpoint the foods that are affecting your gut and eliminate the discomfort they cause. The Complete Low FODMAP Diet for Beginners will guide you step-by-step, helping you identify your triggers, offering personalized dietary solutions, and showing you how to reintroduce foods so you can enjoy life without the burden of digestive stress. With practical advice, clear explanations, and an array of delicious, easy-to-make recipes, you'll have all the tools you need to transform your relationship with food and improve your well-being.

Countless individuals worldwide have found relief and newfound freedom through the Low FODMAP diet. From athletes to busy parents, from professionals to students—those who once felt trapped by their symptoms are now living without fear of food and regaining control over their bodies. The positive impact is undeniable: reduced bloating, less pain, more energy, and an overall better quality of life.

In this book, you'll find not just a diet plan, but a lifestyle change. Inside, you'll discover tailored meal plans to kick start your journey, flavorful recipes to keep your taste buds satisfied, and actionable tips that make living Low FODMAP easy and enjoyable. Whether you're cooking breakfast, preparing snacks, or crafting an indulgent dessert, we've got your digestive health covered.

Are you ready to reclaim your life, find joy in eating again, and say goodbye to the discomfort that has held you back? Take control of your health by following the guidance in The Complete Low FODMAP Diet for Beginners. With practical tools, expert advice, and long-term strategies, this book is your pathway to making lasting, positive changes. It's time to feel good about what you eat—starting today.

CHAPTER ONE

UNDERSTANDING THE LOW FODMAP DIET

The Low FODMAP Diet is an eating plan specifically designed to alleviate symptoms of irritable bowel syndrome (IBS) and other digestive issues by reducing the intake of certain carbohydrates known to trigger symptoms. The concept of FODMAPs, or Fermentable Oligosaccharides, Disaccharides, Monosaccharides, and Polyols, is at the heart of this diet. These carbohydrates are found in many foods, and while they are harmless for most people, they can cause discomfort for those with IBS or other gut sensitivities. The Complete Low FODMAP Diet for Beginners offers a comprehensive guide for understanding and implementing this diet to improve gut health, manage symptoms, and enhance overall well-being.

Understanding FODMAPs

FODMAPs are short-chain carbohydrates and sugar alcohols that can be poorly absorbed in the small intestine. They include:

Fermentable Oligosaccharides These are found in foods like wheat, rye, garlic, and onions.

Disaccharides: Lactose, found in milk and dairy products, falls into this category.

Monosaccharides: Foods high in fructose, such as certain fruits, honey, and high-fructose corn syrup, belong here.

Polyols: These are sugar alcohols found in certain fruits and vegetables and are often used as artificial sweeteners in sugar-free foods.

The digestion of FODMAPs can be problematic for people with IBS or other digestive disorders because they are not easily absorbed by the small intestine. When they reach the colon, they are fermented by bacteria, leading to the production of gas and drawing water into the intestine. This process can lead to common IBS symptoms such as bloating, cramping, diarrhea, constipation, and discomfort.

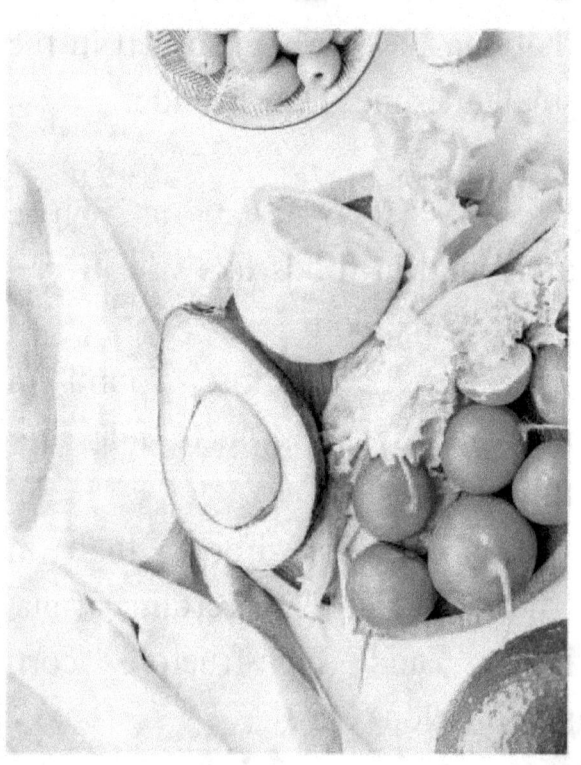

ROLE OF FODMAPS IN GUT HEALTH

The relationship between FODMAPs and gut health is rooted in how the body processes these carbohydrates. In most people, FODMAPs do not cause any issues, but for those with a sensitive digestive system, they can trigger a variety of uncomfortable symptoms. The excess water in the intestines caused by the poor absorption of FODMAPs can lead to diarrhea, while the production of gas from bacterial fermentation can result in bloating and abdominal pain. Additionally, FODMAPs can affect motility, which can either speed up or slow down bowel movements, contributing to either diarrhea or constipation.

By limiting high-FODMAP foods, the goal is to reduce these symptoms and improve the overall quality of life for those who struggle with gut sensitivities. The Complete Low FODMAP Diet for Beginners emphasizes a practical approach to understanding which foods are high or low in FODMAPs, and how to transition to a diet that minimizes their intake.

BASICS OF THE LOW FODMAP DIET

The Low FODMAP Diet consists of three phases, aimed at identifying and managing food triggers:

Elimination Phase: This is the first and most restrictive phase of the diet, where high-FODMAP foods are removed from the diet for a period of 4 to 6 weeks. This phase allows for the reduction of symptoms and provides a clearer understanding of how FODMAPs may be affecting an individual's gut health.

Reintroduction Phase: After the initial period of elimination, FODMAPs are gradually reintroduced, one group at a time, to identify specific triggers. This process helps to understand which types of FODMAPs can be tolerated and in what quantities. It is important to reintroduce foods one at a time to accurately assess their impact on symptoms.

Personalization Phase: This final phase involves establishing a long-term eating plan tailored to an individual's tolerance to FODMAPs. It allows for a balanced and enjoyable diet while managing symptoms effectively.

The diet is not intended to be a permanent exclusion of all high-FODMAP foods. Instead, it is designed to provide a structured approach to identifying personal triggers and developing a sustainable way of eating that minimizes discomfort while ensuring nutritional adequacy.

FODMAPs and IBS: Relief through Diet

For people with IBS, the Low FODMAP Diet can offer significant relief from debilitating symptoms. Studies have shown that up to 75% of those who follow a low FODMAP diet experience a significant improvement in symptoms. By reducing the intake of foods that are poorly absorbed, fermented by gut bacteria, and that can pull excess water into the intestines, the diet can help regulate bowel movements, reduce bloating, and minimize pain and discomfort.

Moreover, The Complete Low FODMAP Diet for Beginners outlines the role of diet in symptom management. It provides clear guidelines on how to identify high-FODMAP foods and replace them with suitable low-FODMAP alternatives. For example, instead of high-FODMAP dairy products like milk, lactose-free options or almond milk can be used. High-FODMAP fruits like apples and pears can be replaced with bananas, blueberries, or strawberries. By understanding these swaps, individuals can enjoy a wide variety of foods while adhering to the principles of the Low FODMAP Diet.

FODMAPs and Other Digestive Issues

While IBS is the most common condition managed with a Low FODMAP Diet, other digestive disorders can also benefit. Conditions like small intestinal bacterial overgrowth (SIBO), functional bloating, and functional diarrhea may also see symptom relief through FODMAP modification. Each condition has unique characteristics, and while the Low FODMAP Diet may not be a cure-all, it can provide an effective strategy for symptom management and quality of life improvement.

It's important to note that the Low FODMAP Diet should be followed under the guidance of a healthcare professional, particularly a dietitian, to ensure that the elimination and reintroduction phases are conducted correctly and that the diet remains balanced and nutritionally adequate.

The Low FODMAP Diet is a scientifically backed approach to managing gut health, particularly for those suffering from IBS and other digestive sensitivities. By understanding and controlling the intake of specific types of carbohydrates, individuals can significantly reduce their symptoms and improve their quality of life.

The Complete Low FODMAP Diet for Beginners serves as a valuable resource, offering practical advice, structured plans, and guidance for those starting on their Low FODMAP journey. With proper understanding and implementation, this diet can make a marked difference in gut health and overall well-being.

THE SCIENCE BEHIND IT: PHASES OF THE LOW FODMAP DIET

The Low FODMAP Diet is rooted in the science of understanding how certain carbohydrates affect gut health. FODMAPs, which stand for Fermentable Oligosaccharides, Disaccharides, Monosaccharides, and Polyols, are types of carbohydrates that are poorly absorbed in the small intestine.

When these carbohydrates reach the large intestine, they are fermented by bacteria, which produces gas.

Additionally, they can draw excess water into the intestines, leading to symptoms such as bloating, abdominal pain, diarrhea, and constipation, particularly in individuals with conditions like IBS (Irritable Bowel Syndrome).

The Science Behind the Low FODMAP Diet

The goal of the Low FODMAP Diet is to reduce or eliminate these troublesome carbohydrates from the diet to lessen the severity of digestive symptoms. The diet works by reducing the intake of FODMAPs, which in turn decreases the fermentation process and water content in the bowel, helping to minimize symptoms of gas, bloating, and irregular bowel movements.

The process is divided into three main phases: Elimination, Reintroduction, and Maintenance (Personalization). Each phase plays a critical role in identifying and managing food triggers.

1. Elimination Phase

The elimination phase is the initial step and typically lasts 4 to 6 weeks. During this period, all high-FODMAP foods are removed from the diet to provide relief from digestive symptoms. High-FODMAP foods include certain fruits (like apples and mangoes), vegetables (like onions and garlic), dairy products (containing lactose), wheat-based products, and certain artificial sweeteners. The aim is to reduce the fermentable carbohydrate load on the gut, thereby minimizing gas production, bloating, and water retention in the intestines.

The science behind this phase is to give the gut a "break" from the substances that tend to provoke symptoms. Many individuals with IBS or other sensitivities will notice significant improvement during this time.

2. Reintroduction Phase

Once symptoms are under control, the reintroduction phase begins. In this phase, FODMAP-containing foods are gradually reintroduced into the diet one at a time. This is done systematically, and each food or group of FODMAPs is tested for tolerance.

For example, an individual might first try reintroducing a food high in oligosaccharides (like wheat) and monitor for any symptoms over a few days before moving on to reintroduce another type of FODMAP (like lactose).

The reintroduction process allows for the identification of specific triggers. This step is important because not all individuals are sensitive to all FODMAPs. By pinpointing which particular FODMAPs cause symptoms, a more tailored and balanced diet can be developed that reduces symptoms while allowing a greater variety of foods.

3. Maintenance (Personalization) Phase

The final phase is maintenance or personalization, where a long-term eating plan is developed based on the individual's specific FODMAP tolerances discovered during the reintroduction phase. The goal here is to maintain symptom control while expanding the variety of foods in the diet to ensure it is balanced and nutritionally complete. Foods that are identified as well-tolerated can be regularly included, while those that trigger symptoms should be minimized or avoided.

This personalized approach is crucial for long-term gut health and overall well-being, as it prevents unnecessary restriction of foods and ensures that the diet remains diverse and enjoyable while still managing digestive symptoms effectively.

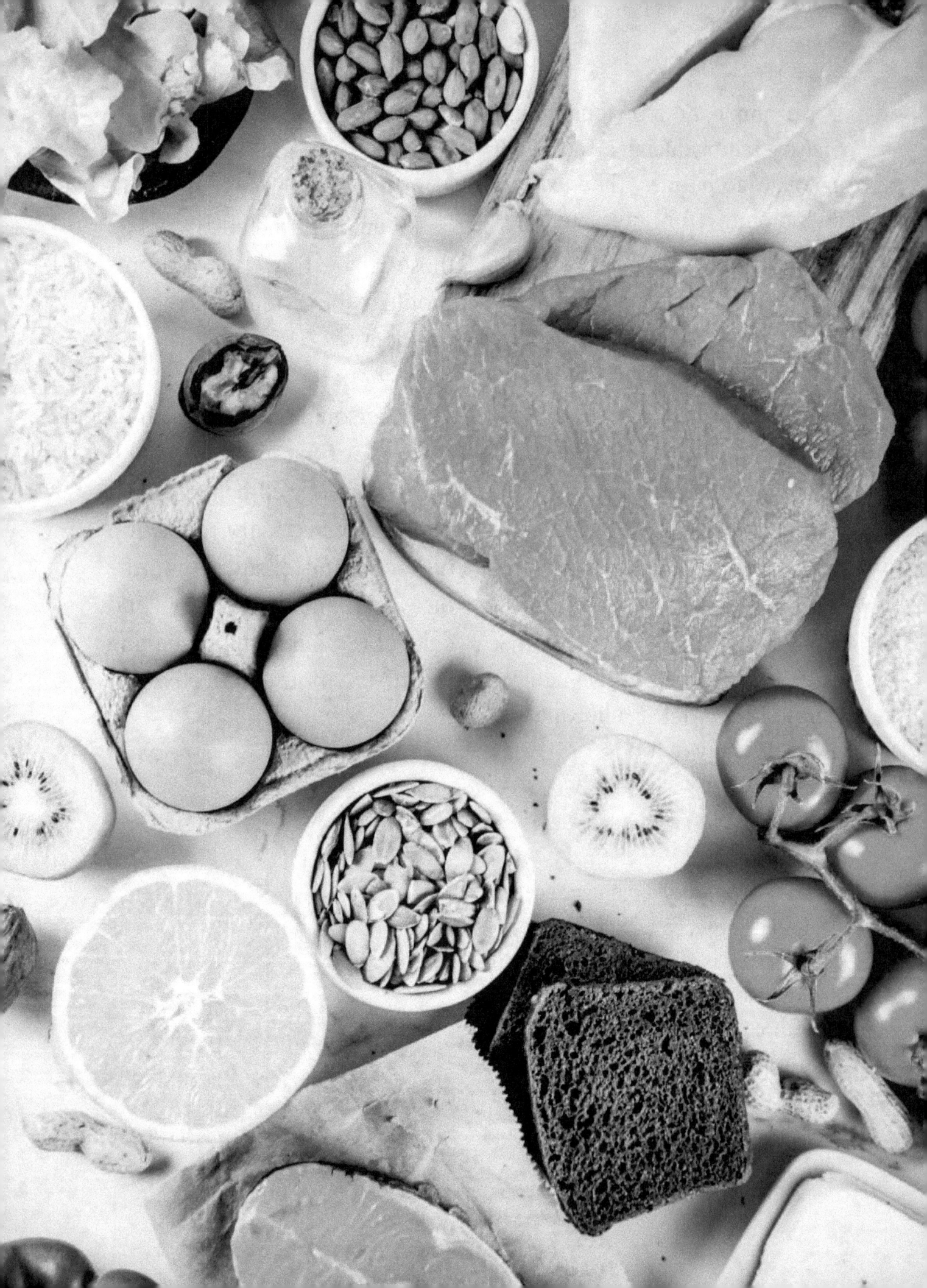

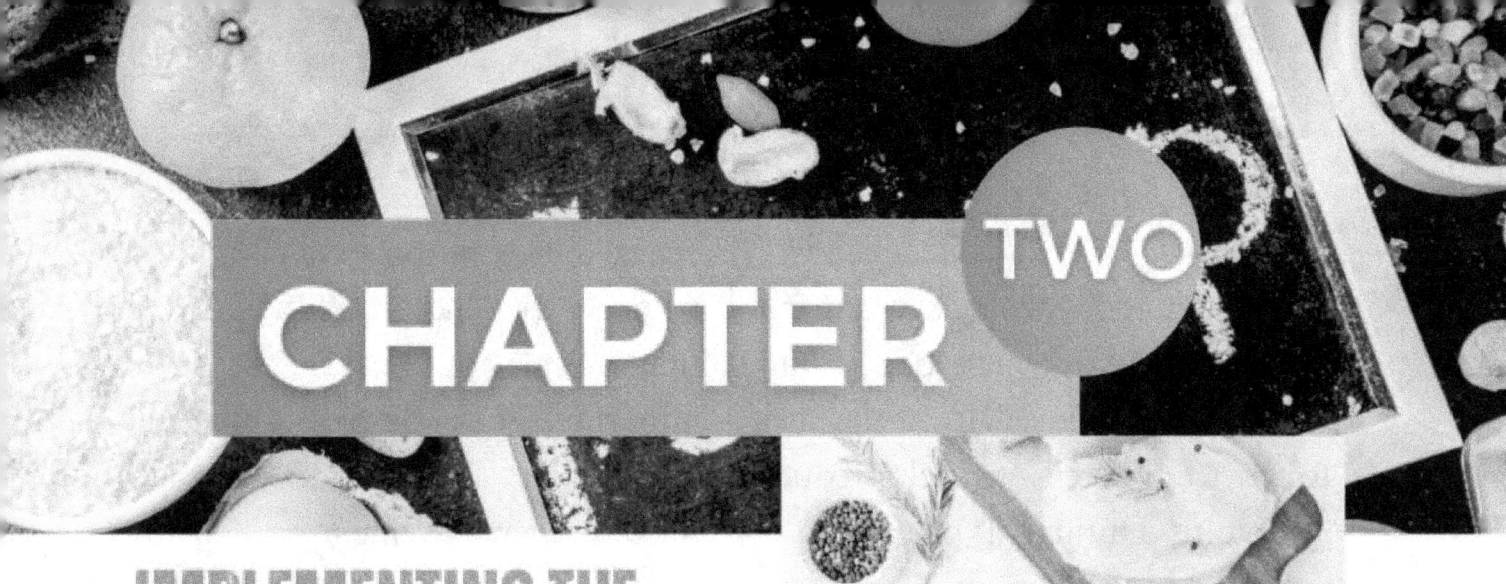

CHAPTER TWO

IMPLEMENTING THE LOW FODMAP DIET

Implementing the Low FODMAP Diet can be highly effective in managing symptoms of IBS and other digestive disorders. The process requires a step-by-step approach that involves identifying triggers, adjusting food choices, and maintaining a balanced diet. Below is a guide on how to effectively implement this diet.

1. Preparation and Planning

Before beginning the Low FODMAP Diet, it is important to gather information, plan meals, and track symptoms. It's recommended to consult with a dietitian or healthcare professional who is familiar with the diet to ensure it is done correctly and to prevent unnecessary nutrient deficiencies. During the preparation phase:

Educate Yourself: Learn about high and low FODMAP foods to identify what needs to be eliminated.

Meal Planning: Create meal plans for the elimination phase to ensure compliance and to ease the transition into the diet.

Symptom Tracking: Keep a food and symptom diary to track any changes in digestive symptoms. This will help identify improvements and better understand how certain foods affect you.

2. Elimination Phase: Reducing High-FODMAP Foods

The elimination phase is where all high-FODMAP foods are temporarily removed from the diet for 4 to 6 weeks to help reduce symptoms. During this phase:

Replace High-FODMAP Foods: Swap out high-FODMAP foods with suitable low-FODMAP alternatives. For example:
Replace onions and garlic with chives or the green part of spring onions.
Use lactose-free milk or almond milk instead of regular cow's milk.
Switch high-FODMAP fruits like apples and pears to low-FODMAP options like strawberries, blueberries, or oranges.
Read Food Labels: Be mindful of ingredients, particularly those containing wheat, high-fructose corn syrup, inulin, or artificial sweeteners ending in "-ol" (e.g., sorbitol, mannitol).

Monitor Symptoms: Track any changes in symptoms closely. Many people experience relief within the first couple of weeks, but it is important to complete the full elimination phase to ensure maximum improvement.

3. Reintroduction Phase: Identifying Triggers

Once symptoms are under control, the next step is to reintroduce high-FODMAP foods one at a time. The purpose is to identify specific triggers while allowing for more food variety in the diet. To do this effectively:

Introduce One Food at a Time: Choose one food high in a specific FODMAP group and introduce it in a small portion (e.g., a few pieces of wheat bread for oligosaccharides or a small amount of milk for lactose). Consume it over a few days while monitoring symptoms.
Increase Serving Size Gradually: If no symptoms are experienced, try increasing the serving size to assess tolerance levels. If symptoms arise, that food may be a trigger, and its intake should be minimized

or monitored.

Track and Record: Continue to use the food diary to record reactions to each food. This will help in clearly identifying which FODMAPs are well-tolerated and which are problematic.

4. Personalization Phase: Creating a Sustainable Long-Term Plan

The personalization phase is about building a balanced diet that minimizes symptoms while allowing as much variety as possible. This phase is important to ensure that the diet is nutritionally adequate and sustainable over time. To maintain this phase:

Develop a Balanced Diet: Focus on including a variety of tolerated low- and moderate-FODMAP foods to cover all essential nutrients.

Reintroduce Well-Tolerated Foods Regularly: If certain high-FODMAP foods are found to be well-tolerated, incorporate them back into regular meals to ensure a wide range of nutrients and to avoid unnecessary restrictions.

Adjust as Needed: The Low FODMAP Diet is dynamic. Your tolerance to certain foods may change over time, so it's important to be flexible and adjust your diet as necessary.

5. Practical Tips for Success

Implementing the Low FODMAP Diet may seem challenging initially, but the following practical tips can aid in maintaining the diet effectively:

Prepare Meals at Home: Preparing meals from scratch allows you to control the ingredients and avoid hidden high-FODMAP components.

Use Low-FODMAP Cookbooks or Apps: There are various resources available with low-FODMAP recipes, meal plans, and guidance on food choices, which can be helpful for meal preparation and variety.

Plan for Dining Out: When eating out, plan ahead by checking restaurant menus online and choosing dishes that are more likely to be low in FODMAPs. Don't hesitate to ask for modifications or to inquire about ingredients in meals.

Stay Hydrated and Exercise: Supporting your digestive system also involves drinking plenty of water and staying active, as both can help improve digestion and manage IBS symptoms.

6. Monitoring and Ongoing Support

Adopting the Low FODMAP Diet is a process that requires ongoing monitoring and potential adjustments. Regular follow-up with a dietitian or healthcare professional is beneficial for:

Nutritional Guidance: To ensure you're getting all the essential nutrients, especially during the elimination phase where certain food groups are limited.

Symptom Management: To assess symptom progression and make necessary changes to the diet for long-term effectiveness.

Emotional Support: For some, adjusting to the Low FODMAP Diet can be a significant lifestyle change. Professional support can help in navigating challenges and staying motivated.

Implementing the Low FODMAP Diet can significantly improve the quality of life for individuals suffering from IBS or other digestive issues. Through careful planning, tracking, and professional guidance, individuals can effectively manage symptoms, discover personal food triggers, and develop a balanced, enjoyable, and sustainable eating plan tailored to their needs.

BENEFITS AND GOALS

Following the Low FODMAP Diet can offer significant benefits, particularly for individuals dealing with IBS (Irritable Bowel Syndrome) or other functional gastrointestinal disorders. By eliminating certain carbohydrates that can contribute to digestive discomfort, the diet aims to improve quality of life, reduce digestive symptoms, and support better overall gut health. Here's a breakdown of the primary benefits and goals of following the Low FODMAP Diet:

Benefits of the Low FODMAP Diet

Symptom Relief for IBS and Digestive Disorders

The main benefit of the Low FODMAP Diet is the reduction of uncomfortable digestive symptoms such as bloating, gas, abdominal pain, diarrhea, and constipation. For individuals with IBS, adhering to this diet can alleviate these symptoms by reducing the intake of foods that are poorly digested and cause fermentation in the gut.

Better Gut Health and Improved Digestion

By reducing high-FODMAP foods that are known to contribute to digestive discomfort, the diet can help to balance gut bacteria and enhance digestion. Individuals often report feeling lighter and more comfortable, with a reduction in bloating and abdominal distension.

Personalized Understanding of Food Triggers

A major advantage of the Low FODMAP Diet is that it allows individuals to pinpoint their specific food triggers through the reintroduction phase. This knowledge empowers them to make informed food choices, knowing what to eat and what to avoid to prevent symptoms.

Enhanced Quality of Life

Alleviating the symptoms of IBS or other digestive issues often leads to an improved overall quality of life. Many people experience better mental health, increased energy levels, and greater social freedom as they no longer have to worry about sudden discomfort or digestive emergencies.

Increased Variety and Flexibility Over Time

While the elimination phase is restrictive, the long-term goal is to reintroduce well-tolerated foods back into the diet, creating a personalized and balanced eating plan. This helps ensure that individuals are not unnecessarily cutting out entire food groups, leading to a more flexible and enjoyable way of eating.

Potential Support for Other Health Conditions

Although primarily used for IBS, research suggests that the Low FODMAP Diet may also help manage symptoms in other conditions, such as inflammatory bowel disease (IBD), functional bloating, small intestinal bacterial overgrowth (SIBO), and functional dyspepsia. However, it is important to follow this diet under medical supervision when dealing with other health conditions.

Goals of Following the Low FODMAP Diet

Symptom Management and Control

The main goal of the Low FODMAP Diet is to manage and reduce the frequency and severity of digestive symptoms. By identifying and reducing FODMAP intake, individuals aim to control symptoms like bloating, gas, abdominal pain, and irregular bowel movements that are associated with IBS and other gut issues.

Personalized Diet and Symptom Awareness

A key objective of the diet is to help individuals understand their own food sensitivities through careful reintroduction and monitoring. This tailored approach allows for a more personalized diet that is not only effective in symptom relief but also balanced in terms of nutrition.

Restoring Digestive Comfort and Balance

Another goal is to create a sense of digestive comfort by reducing foods that ferment rapidly and draw excess water into the intestines, which can lead to discomfort. By reducing these "triggers," the diet helps restore normal digestion and gut function.

Long-Term Lifestyle and Nutritional Balance

The Low FODMAP Diet aims to be sustainable for the long term, allowing individuals to reintroduce tolerable foods and maintain a balanced, nutritionally adequate diet. The ultimate goal is to help people develop a diverse and flexible eating pattern that supports both their digestive health and overall nutritional needs.

Empowerment and Control Over Eating Habits

Following the Low FODMAP Diet can help individuals gain control over their food choices and reduce anxiety around eating. Understanding which foods trigger symptoms can empower people to make dietary decisions that support their health and well-being, leading to more confidence in social situations involving food.

Improving Mental and Emotional Health

Digestive symptoms can significantly impact mental and emotional health, contributing to stress, anxiety, and a reduced sense of well-being. By managing symptoms through the Low FODMAP Diet, individuals often experience not only physical relief but also an improvement in mood, less anxiety around food, and better mental health.

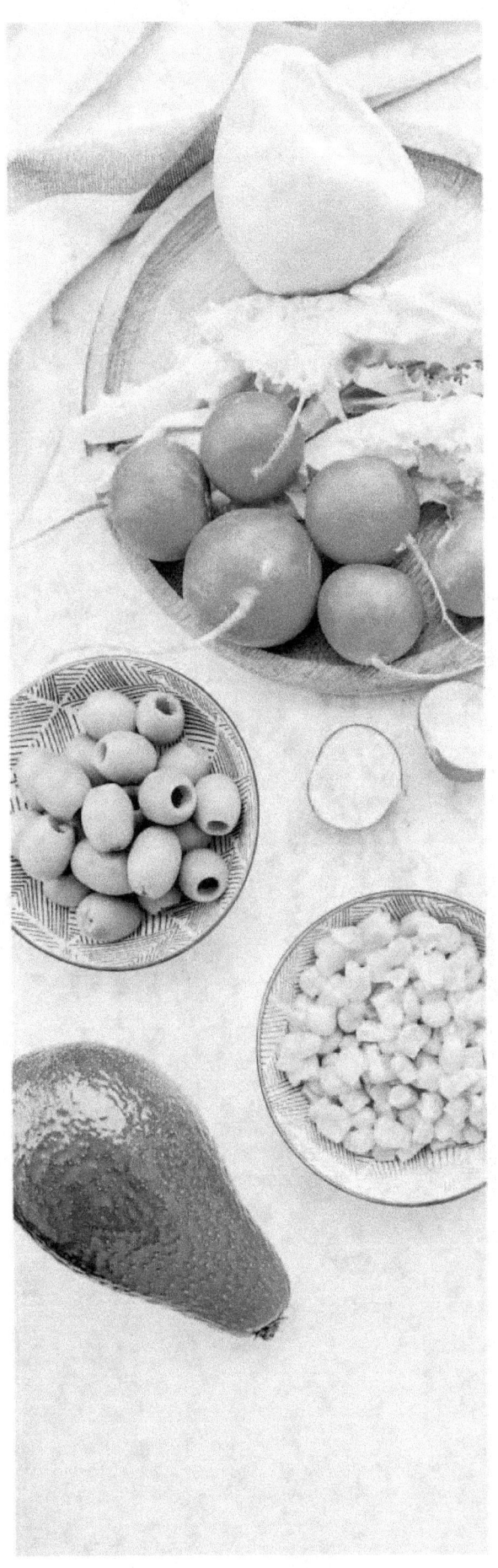

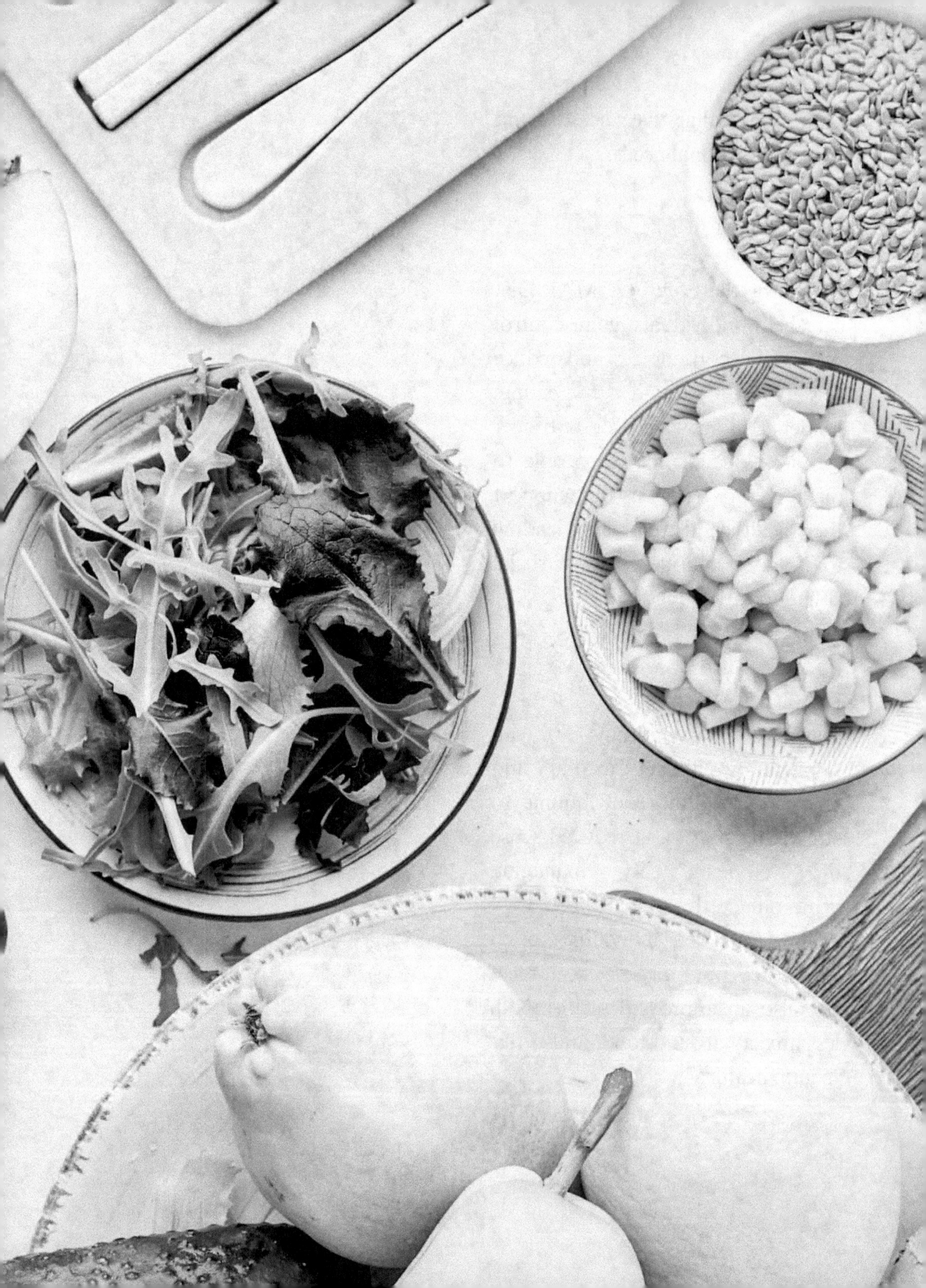

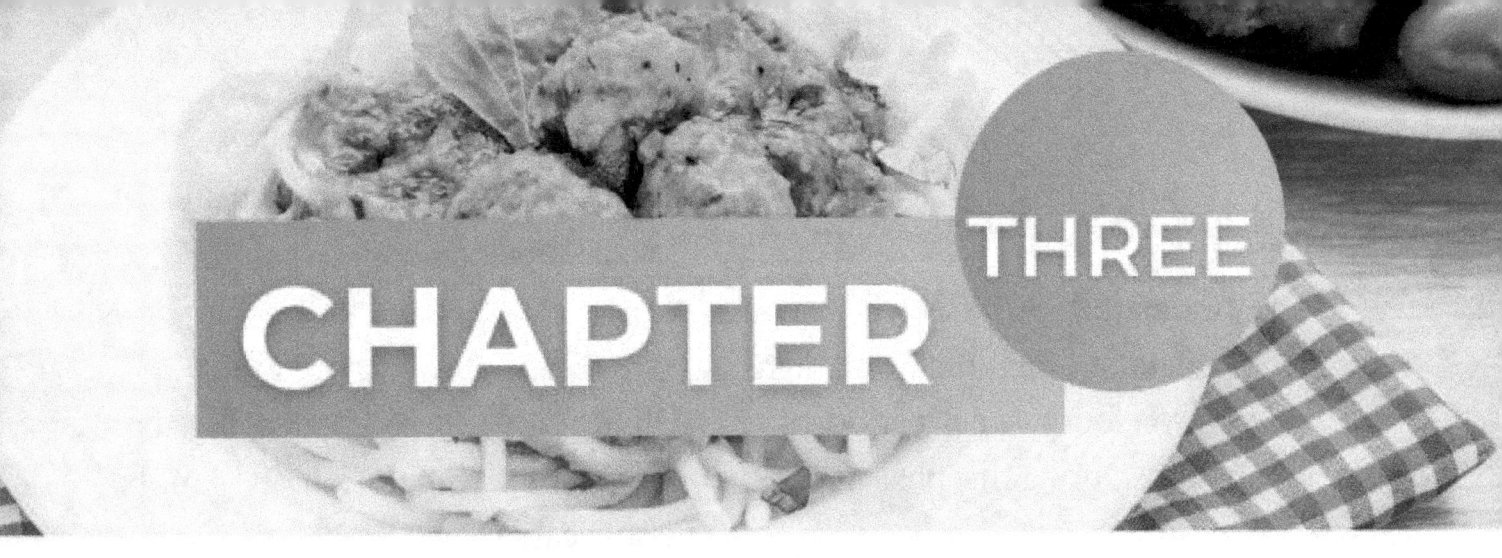

CHAPTER THREE

PUTTING THE LOW FODMAP DIET INTO PRACTICE

Putting the Low FODMAP Diet into practice involves several key steps that help you transition from your current eating habits to a more symptom-managed lifestyle. This process can be manageable and rewarding when approached with the right strategies. Here's how to effectively implement the Low FODMAP Diet and make it a part of your daily routine:

Step 1: Start with Preparation

Preparation is essential for successfully putting the Low FODMAP Diet into practice. Since it involves eliminating certain foods that you might regularly consume, it helps to plan ahead.

Educate Yourself: Learn about which foods are high and low in FODMAPs. A variety of books, apps, and resources can provide lists of foods to include and avoid.

Meal Planning and Grocery Shopping: Plan your meals and snacks for the week. Make a grocery list based on low FODMAP foods, such as meat, fish, eggs, firm tofu, gluten-free grains (like rice, oats, and quinoa), and low-FODMAP fruits and vegetables (e.g., strawberries, carrots, spinach).

Clear Out Your Pantry: Remove or set aside high-FODMAP foods, including products that contain wheat, onion, garlic, certain dairy products, and artificial sweeteners ending in "-ol" like sorbitol or xylitol. Stock up on low-FODMAP staples.

Step 2: Begin the Elimination Phase

The elimination phase is where you start reducing your intake of high-FODMAP foods for a period of 4 to 6 weeks. During this phase:

Keep Meals Simple: Stick to plain and minimally processed foods that are low in FODMAPs, such as grilled meats or fish, eggs, potatoes, zucchini, lettuce, and gluten-free pasta. This simplicity helps you easily monitor symptoms and avoid accidentally consuming high-FODMAP ingredients.

Find Suitable Substitutes: Swap high-FODMAP ingredients with low-FODMAP alternatives. For example:

Replace milk with lactose-free milk or almond milk.

Use green tops of scallions or chives in place of onion.

Use herbs and spices to add flavor to meals instead of garlic (garlic-infused oil is a flavorful alternative that is low in FODMAPs).

Track Your Progress: Keep a food and symptom journal to track how each meal affects your digestion. Note any patterns that might indicate improvement or trigger foods.

Step 3: Navigate Eating Out

Dining out can be challenging, but with some preparation, it can be manageable.

Choose the Right Restaurant: Opt for restaurants that have gluten-free or customizable menu options. Steakhouses, seafood places, or restaurants offering simple grilled meats and vegetables are often good choices.

Plan Ahead: Check menus online before going out and call the restaurant to ask about ingredients and possible modifications to dishes.

Communicate Clearly: Politely inform the server about your dietary needs. Ask for meals to be prepared without sauces, dressings, or added ingredients that might contain high-FODMAP elements.

Step 4: Enter the Reintroduction Phase

Once your symptoms are under control during the elimination phase, you'll move on to the reintroduction phase to identify specific FODMAP triggers. This phase requires patience and careful testing:

Test Foods One at a Time: Start by reintroducing a small amount of a food that contains a specific type of FODMAP (e.g., reintroducing wheat for oligosaccharides or milk for lactose). Test the food for 3-4 days, gradually increasing the amount.

Monitor Symptoms Carefully: Record any reactions in your journal, such as bloating, gas, or changes in bowel movements. If symptoms reappear, the tested food may be a trigger, and its intake should be minimized.

Proceed with Caution: After testing one type of FODMAP, move on to another food type (e.g., fructose, polyols) until you have identified your personal triggers and tolerances.

Step 5: Establish the Maintenance (Personalization) Phase

The final step of implementing the Low FODMAP Diet is creating a balanced, long-term eating plan based on your reintroduction results. This personalized phase focuses on managing symptoms while maintaining a nutritionally complete diet.

Balance Low and Tolerated High-FODMAP Foods: Incorporate a wide variety of tolerated low-FODMAP foods and the specific high-FODMAP foods that you can handle. Aim to have a balanced intake of protein, carbohydrates, fruits, vegetables, and healthy fats.

Experiment with Recipes: Once you know which foods work for you, expand your diet with creative low-FODMAP recipes. Experiment with flavors, spices, and cooking methods to make meals enjoyable.

Reevaluate Over Time: Food tolerances can change over time, so periodically test certain foods again to see if you have developed a greater tolerance, or if other foods have become less manageable.

Step 6: Tips for Ongoing Success

To maintain a Low FODMAP lifestyle, the following tips can support your journey:

Stay Hydrated: Drink plenty of water throughout the day to support digestion and prevent constipation, especially if your diet is high in fiber.

Choose Whole Foods: Focus on minimally processed foods like fresh vegetables, fruits, lean proteins, and whole grains. Avoid packaged foods with hidden high-FODMAP ingredients.

Listen to Your Body: Be mindful of how you feel after eating different foods. Your body can guide you in making better choices and adjusting your diet as needed.

Step 7: Seek Support and Community

Since the Low FODMAP Diet can be challenging to navigate alone, having support is invaluable:

Work with a Dietitian: A dietitian knowledgeable in the Low FODMAP Diet can provide meal ideas, troubleshoot challenges, and ensure that you're meeting your nutritional needs.

Join Support Groups: Online forums, social media groups, and local support communities can be great resources for recipe ideas, product recommendations, and encouragement.

LOW FODMAP LIFESTYLE AND DIGESTIVE HEALTH TIPS

Adopting a Low FODMAP lifestyle can greatly improve digestive health and help manage conditions like IBS (Irritable Bowel Syndrome). Here are some practical tips to support your journey in maintaining a low FODMAP lifestyle while ensuring your digestive system stays healthy and well-balanced:

1. Build Balanced Low FODMAP Meals

When following a Low FODMAP lifestyle, it's important to include balanced meals that support your digestive health:

Balance Protein, Carbohydrates, and Fats: Include a variety of low FODMAP proteins (chicken, beef, fish, eggs, tofu), carbs (rice, potatoes, gluten-free grains), and healthy fats (olive oil, nuts like walnuts, chia seeds).

Incorporate Fiber-Rich Foods: While certain fibers are high in FODMAPs, many low-FODMAP options like oats, chia seeds, flaxseeds, and kiwi can help improve digestion, support regular bowel movements, and reduce symptoms of constipation.

Include Probiotic-Rich Foods: Probiotics are beneficial for gut health as they support the balance of good bacteria in your gut. Low-FODMAP options include lactose-free yogurt, kefir (lactose-free), and fermented foods like pickles or kimchi (in small amounts).

2. Practice Mindful Eating

Mindful eating can play a key role in improving digestion and reducing symptoms:

Eat Slowly and Chew Thoroughly: Eating slowly and chewing well helps break down food more effectively, easing the burden on your digestive system.

Avoid Overeating: Consuming large portions can overwhelm your gut and lead to bloating and discomfort. Try eating smaller, more frequent meals throughout the day to ease digestion.

Listen to Your Hunger Cues: Eating when you're genuinely hungry and stopping when you're comfortably full can prevent overeating and support better digestion.

3. Stay Hydrated

Proper hydration is crucial for digestive health:

Drink Enough Water: Aim to drink at least 8 cups of water per day to aid digestion, support bowel regularity, and prevent dehydration.

Spread Fluid Intake Throughout the Day: Sipping on water or herbal teas throughout the day, instead of consuming large amounts at once, can help prevent bloating and facilitate digestion.

4. Exercise Regularly for Gut Health

Physical activity helps maintain healthy digestion and can improve IBS symptoms:

Incorporate Gentle Movement: Activities like walking, yoga, and stretching can help stimulate digestion, reduce bloating, and ease constipation.

Avoid Intense Workouts Immediately After Meals: Engaging in strenuous exercise right after eating can disrupt digestion. It's best to allow time for your food to settle before engaging in high-intensity activities.

5. Manage Stress and Mental Well-being

Stress and anxiety can exacerbate digestive symptoms, especially for those with IBS:

Practice Relaxation Techniques: Mindfulness, meditation, deep breathing, and progressive muscle relaxation are helpful ways to manage stress, which in turn can ease digestive discomfort.

Engage in Hobbies and Activities You Enjoy: Whether it's reading, gardening, or spending time with loved ones, doing things that make you happy can help reduce stress and promote a more relaxed digestive system.

6. Maintain a Food and Symptom Journal

Tracking your food intake and symptoms can help identify triggers and support better food choices:

Record Meals and Snacks: Keep a daily record of what you eat, portion sizes, and the timing of meals.

Note Digestive Symptoms and Patterns: Track how you feel after meals, noting any discomfort, bloating, bowel changes, or other symptoms. This can help pinpoint specific foods or behaviors that affect your digestion.

7. Make Smart Substitutions and Meal Prep

Managing a Low FODMAP lifestyle is easier when you prepare and make smart substitutions:

Use Low-FODMAP Swaps: Opt for gluten-free bread and pasta, lactose-free dairy products, and low-FODMAP fruits (like strawberries, oranges, and bananas) instead of high-FODMAP ones.

Batch Cooking and Meal Prep: Preparing meals in advance helps you stay on track and reduces the likelihood of accidentally consuming high-FODMAP foods when you're short on time.

8. Eat Low-FODMAP Snacks
Snacking is a great way to prevent overeating during meals and stabilize your energy levels:

Choose Gut-Friendly Snacks: Low-FODMAP snack options include rice cakes with peanut butter, lactose-free yogurt with berries, veggie sticks with hummus (low-FODMAP), or a handful of low-FODMAP nuts like walnuts.
Carry Snacks on the Go: Having portable low-FODMAP snacks can help you avoid high-FODMAP foods when you're away from home or in a situation with limited food options.

9. Avoid Gut Irritants
Certain behaviors and foods can irritate your gut, so it's best to minimize or avoid them:

Limit Alcohol, Caffeine, and Carbonated Drinks: These can stimulate or irritate the gut, leading to bloating, gas, and other symptoms. Stick to herbal teas, lactose-free milk, or water.
Be Mindful of Artificial Sweeteners: Sugar alcohols like sorbitol, mannitol, and xylitol are high in FODMAPs and can trigger digestive symptoms.

10. Gradually Increase Fiber with Tolerance
Fiber is important for digestive health but can be problematic in large quantities:

Increase Fiber Slowly: Gradually introduce low-FODMAP fiber sources into your diet to prevent symptoms like bloating and gas.
Pair Fiber with Fluids: Drinking plenty of water alongside fiber-rich foods supports smooth digestion and can prevent constipation.

11. Adjust and Reevaluate Your Diet Regularly
Your body and tolerance levels may change over time, so it's important to be flexible:

Reassess Your Tolerances Periodically: You may find that over time, certain high-FODMAP foods can be better tolerated in small amounts.

Stay Open to Reintroductions: As your digestive health improves, you may want to reintroduce and test new foods occasionally to expand your diet.

CHAPTER FOUR

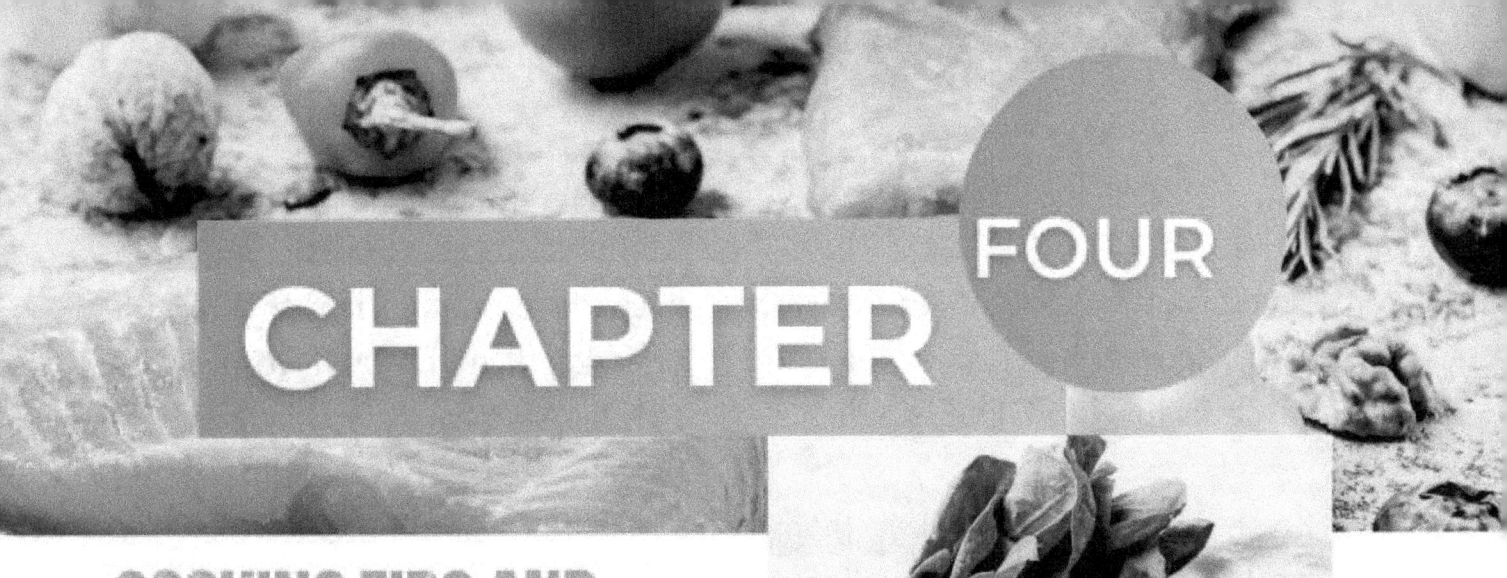

COOKING TIPS AND MODIFICATION

Cooking while following a Low FODMAP Diet requires some adjustments to traditional recipes, but it can still be flavorful and satisfying. Below are practical cooking tips and modifications to help you prepare tasty low FODMAP meals while minimizing digestive discomfort.

1. Replace High FODMAP Ingredients with Low FODMAP Alternatives

Use Garlic and Onion Substitutes: Garlic and onion are high in FODMAPs and often the cause of digestive discomfort. Instead:

Use garlic-infused oil (made by infusing oil with garlic cloves and then removing the cloves) to add flavor without the FODMAPs.

Try the green tops of scallions or chives for an onion-like flavor.

Use spices like cumin, coriander, and asafoetida powder (also called "hing") as flavor boosters.

Swap Dairy Products with Lactose-Free Versions: Many dairy products contain lactose, which is high in FODMAPs.

Use lactose-free milk, yogurt, and cheese as substitutes for regular dairy.

Non-dairy alternatives like almond milk, coconut yogurt, and oat milk (in small amounts) are low in FODMAPs.

2. Use Low-FODMAP Herbs and Spices for Flavor

Enhance the taste of your dishes with herbs and spices that are naturally low in FODMAPs.

Fresh Herbs: Use parsley, thyme, basil, oregano, rosemary, cilantro, mint, and dill to add depth and freshness to your meals.

Dried Spices: Cumin, paprika, turmeric, chili powder, and ginger are great for adding flavor without triggering symptoms.

Flavor Boosters: Lemon or lime juice, vinegars (balsamic, red wine, apple cider), soy sauce (in small quantities), and mustard are safe to use in low FODMAP cooking.

3. Modify Cooking Methods to Suit the Low FODMAP Lifestyle

Certain cooking techniques can help enhance flavors and textures without the need for high FODMAP ingredients.

Roasting Vegetables: Roasting low-FODMAP vegetables like carrots, zucchini, bell peppers, and potatoes brings out their natural sweetness and enhances flavor.

Grilling or Baking Meats and Fish: Marinate meats or fish in lemon juice, olive oil, and herbs, then grill or bake them for a flavorful, low FODMAP meal.

Sautéing with Infused Oils: Using garlic- or herb-infused oils for sautéing meats, vegetables, or grains adds flavor without the digestive discomfort caused by high-FODMAP garlic or onion.

4. Use Low-FODMAP Thickeners and Binders

High-FODMAP ingredients like wheat flour, cornstarch, or cream are often used as thickeners in sauces and soups. Try these low-FODMAP alternatives:

Arrowroot or Tapioca Starch: These can be used as thickening agents for sauces, soups, and gravies.

Gluten-Free Flour Blends: Use blends made from rice, potato, or quinoa flour for baking or as a thickener.

Coconut Cream or Lactose-Free Cream: Use these for creamy soups, sauces, or desserts as a replacement for regular cream.

5. Modify High-FODMAP Recipes to Make Them Friendly

You can make your favorite high-FODMAP recipes suitable for your low FODMAP lifestyle with simple modifications.

Soups and Stews: Use a vegetable stock made without onion or garlic, or make your own low-FODMAP broth using carrots, celery, herbs, and spices.

Pasta and Rice Dishes: Choose gluten-free pasta made from rice or quinoa, and replace regular pasta sauces with low-FODMAP tomato-based sauces flavored with herbs and spices.

Baked Goods: For baked goods like muffins, cookies, or bread, use low-FODMAP flours like almond flour, rice flour, or a gluten-free blend, and swap out high-FODMAP sweeteners for maple syrup or brown sugar.

6. Watch Serving Sizes for FODMAP-Friendly Ingredients

Some ingredients are low in FODMAPs when consumed in small amounts but can become high in FODMAPs when larger quantities are eaten.

Stick to Recommended Portions: For example, a small amount of sweet potato (1/2 cup) is considered low FODMAP, but larger portions may trigger symptoms. Be mindful of serving sizes to stay within low-FODMAP limits.

Mix and Match: Combine a variety of low-FODMAP vegetables in your meals, such as carrots, zucchini, green beans, and spinach, to create balance and variety without overloading on any single ingredient.

7. Use Low-FODMAP Sweeteners and Flavorings

Some common sweeteners like honey, high-fructose corn syrup, and agave are high in FODMAPs. Use these alternatives to add sweetness without causing discomfort:

Maple Syrup and Table Sugar: Both are considered low in FODMAPs and can be used in small amounts to sweeten dishes.

Vanilla Extract and Cocoa Powder: Use these to add flavor to desserts, smoothies, or baked goods without adding FODMAPs.

Stevia and Monk Fruit: These are low-FODMAP sweeteners and suitable substitutes for sugar or other high-FODMAP sweeteners.

8. Use Gut-Friendly Cooking Methods

Low-FODMAP cooking involves methods that support digestion and make food more gut-friendly.

Slow Cooking and Braising: Slow cooking lean meats and low-FODMAP vegetables helps break down fibers, making them easier to digest.

Steaming or Boiling: Steaming or boiling vegetables can make them softer and easier on the digestive system.

Pressure Cooking: Pressure cooking can break down fibrous parts of foods and reduce cooking time, which can help those with sensitive digestion.

9. Prepare Batch Meals for Convenience

Preparing low-FODMAP meals in batches can save time and help you stick to the diet.

Cook and Freeze in Portions: Make large batches of soups, stews, or casseroles and freeze them in individual portions for easy, ready-to-eat low-FODMAP meals.

Pre-Cut Vegetables and Meats: Keep low-FODMAP vegetables and proteins pre-cut and portioned in the fridge, so you can quickly assemble salads, stir-fries, or snacks when you're hungry.

10. Use Low-FODMAP Condiments and Sauces

Condiments can make meals more flavorful, but many are high in FODMAPs. Instead, use:

Mustard, Mayonnaise (without added garlic/onion), and Pesto (without garlic): These are flavorful condiments that are generally low in FODMAPs.

Low-FODMAP Tomato Sauces: Make or buy tomato sauces without onion and garlic. Flavor them

with basil, oregano, or other low-FODMAP herbs.
Soy Sauce (in Small Amounts): Soy sauce can be used in moderation. Tamari (a gluten-free soy sauce) is a great alternative.

11. Check Labels for Hidden High-FODMAP Ingredients

Many packaged foods contain hidden FODMAPs, so always check labels:

Avoid Ingredients like "Inulin," "Fructans," "High-Fructose Corn Syrup," and "Sorbitol." These are common high-FODMAP additives found in packaged products.

Look for Certified Low-FODMAP Products: Some brands offer certified low-FODMAP products, which make it easier to incorporate them into your diet without worrying about ingredient triggers.

By following these cooking tips and modifications, you can enjoy flavorful, diverse, and satisfying meals while maintaining a Low FODMAP lifestyle. With practice, preparing low-FODMAP meals will become second nature, helping you manage digestive symptoms while still enjoying your favorite foods.

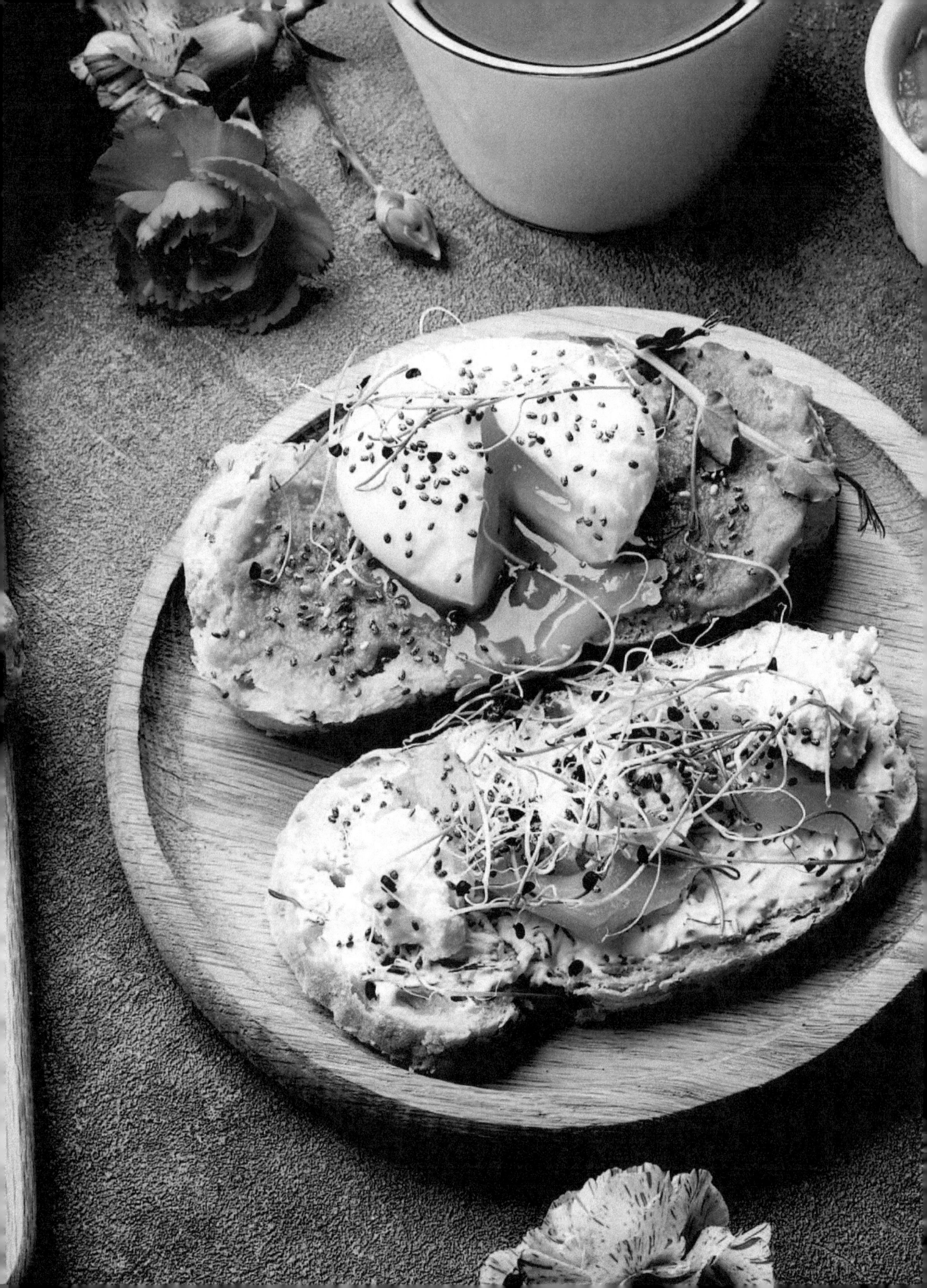

Breakfast Recipes

SCRAMBLED EGGS WITH SPINACH AND TOMATOES

(Serves 2 | 10 mins)

INGREDIENTS

- 4 large eggs
- 1 cup fresh spinach leaves
- 1 medium tomato (diced)
- 1 tbsp olive oil
- Salt and pepper to taste

DIRECTIONS

1. Heat olive oil in a pan over medium heat.
2. Add diced tomatoes and cook until slightly softened.
3. Stir in spinach until wilted.
4. Whisk eggs with salt and pepper in a bowl.
5. Pour eggs into the pan, stirring gently until cooked.
6. Serve warm.

NUTRITIONAL INFO

- Calories: 160
- Protein: 12g
- Fat: 11g
- Carbs: 3g

BANANA ALMOND SMOOTHIE

(Serves 1 | 5 mins)

INGREDIENTS

- 1 ripe banana
- 1 cup almond milk (unsweetened)
- 1 tbsp almond butter
- 1 tsp maple syrup (optional)

DIRECTIONS

1. Place all ingredients in a blender.
2. Blend until smooth and creamy.
3. Taste and add maple syrup if needed.
4. Pour into a glass and serve immediately.

NUTRITIONAL INFO

- Calories: 200
- Protein: 5g
- Fat: 9g
- Carbs: 25g

OATMEAL WITH BLUEBERRIES AND CINNAMON

(Serves 1 | 10 mins)

INGREDIENTS

- 1/2 cup gluten-free oats
- 1 cup water or lactose-free milk
- 1/4 cup fresh blueberries
- 1/4 tsp ground cinnamon

DIRECTIONS

1. In a pot, combine oats and water/milk.
2. Bring to a boil, then reduce to a simmer.
3. Cook for 5-7 minutes, stirring occasionally.
4. Stir in cinnamon.
5. Serve topped with blueberries.
6. Enjoy warm.

NUTRITIONAL INFO

- Calories: 150
- Protein: 4g
- Fat: 3g
- Carbs: 27g

LACTOSE-FREE YOGURT PARFAIT

(Serves 1 | 5 mins)

INGREDIENTS

- 1 cup lactose-free yogurt
- 1/4 cup strawberries (sliced)
- 2 tbsp gluten-free granola
- 1 tsp chia seeds

DIRECTIONS

1. Layer half the yogurt in a bowl or jar.
2. Add half the strawberries and granola.
3. Repeat with remaining yogurt, strawberries, and granola.
4. Sprinkle chia seeds on top.
5. Serve immediately.

NUTRITIONAL INFO

- Calories: 200
- Protein: 6g
- Fat: 5g
- Carbs: 35g

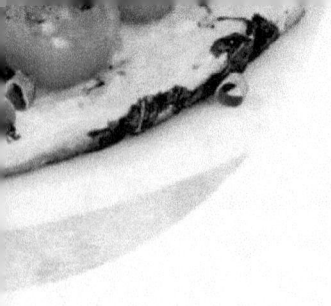

SPINACH AND CHEESE OMELET

(Serves 1 | 10 mins)

INGREDIENTS

- 2 large eggs
- 1/2 cup fresh spinach leaves
- 1/4 cup grated cheddar cheese (lactose-free)
- 1 tbsp olive oil
- Salt and pepper to taste

DIRECTIONS

1. Whisk eggs with salt and pepper in a bowl.
2. Heat olive oil in a pan over medium heat.
3. Pour eggs into the pan, cook until edges set.
4. Add spinach and cheese on half the omelet.
5. Fold the omelet over and cook until cheese melts.
6. Serve warm.

NUTRITIONAL INFO

- Calories: 250
- Protein: 16g
- Fat: 20g
- Carbs: 2g

PEANUT BUTTER RICE CAKES

(Serves 1 | 5 mins)

INGREDIENTS

- 2 rice cakes (plain)
- 2 tbsp natural peanut butter
- 1/2 banana (sliced)

DIRECTIONS

1. Spread peanut butter evenly over each rice cake.
2. Top with banana slices.
3. Optional: drizzle with a tiny bit of maple syrup.
4. Serve immediately.

NUTRITIONAL INFO

- Calories: 220
- Protein: 7g
- Fat: 12g
- Carbs: 25g

QUINOA BREAKFAST BOWL

(Serves 2 | 15 mins)

INGREDIENTS

- 1/2 cup cooked quinoa
- 1 cup lactose-free milk
- 1 tbsp maple syrup
- 1/4 cup blueberries
- 1 tbsp pumpkin seeds

DIRECTIONS

1. Heat cooked quinoa and milk in a pot over medium heat.
2. Stir in maple syrup and simmer for 5 minutes.
3. Divide into bowls.
4. Top with blueberries and pumpkin seeds.
5. Serve warm.

NUTRITIONAL INFO

- Calories: 180
- Protein: 6g
- Fat: 4g
- Carbs: 30g

COCONUT CHIA PUDDING

(Serves 2 | 5 mins prep + 4 hrs chilling)

INGREDIENTS

- 1 cup coconut milk (canned, low-fat)
- 2 tbsp chia seeds
- 1 tbsp maple syrup
- 1/4 cup fresh raspberries

DIRECTIONS

1. In a bowl, mix coconut milk, chia seeds, and maple syrup.
2. Stir well and let sit for 5 minutes.
3. Stir again to prevent clumping.
4. Cover and refrigerate for at least 4 hours (or overnight).
5. Top with raspberries before serving.

NUTRITIONAL INFO

- Calories: 150
- Protein: 2g
- Fat: 12g
- Carbs: 10g

TOMATO AND BASIL FRITTATA

(Serves 3 | 20 mins)

INGREDIENTS

- 6 large eggs
- 1/2 cup diced tomatoes (seeded)
- 1/4 cup lactose-free cheddar cheese
- Fresh basil leaves (chopped)
- 1 tbsp olive oil
- Salt and pepper to taste

DIRECTIONS

1. Preheat oven to 375°F (190°C).
2. In a bowl, whisk eggs, salt, and pepper.
3. Heat oil in an oven-safe pan over medium heat.
4. Pour egg mixture, add tomatoes, cheese, and basil.
5. Cook until edges set, then transfer to the oven.
6. Bake for 10-12 minutes or until fully cooked.

NUTRITIONAL INFO

- Calories: 140
- Protein: 10g
- Fat: 9g
- Carbs: 3g

PUMPKIN SPICE OVERNIGHT OATS

(Serves 1 | 5 mins prep + overnight)

INGREDIENTS

- 1/2 cup gluten-free oats
- 1/2 cup lactose-free milk
- 2 tbsp pumpkin puree (canned, unsweetened)
- 1/2 tsp cinnamon
- 1 tbsp maple syrup

DIRECTIONS

1. In a jar, mix oats, milk, pumpkin puree, cinnamon, and maple syrup.
2. Stir well to combine.
3. Cover and refrigerate overnight.
4. In the morning, stir again and serve cold or warm.

NUTRITIONAL INFO

- Calories: 180
- Protein: 5g
- Fat: 3g
- Carbs: 33g

AVOCADO TOAST WITH POACHED EGG

(Serves 1 | 10 mins)

INGREDIENTS

- 1 slice gluten-free bread, toasted
- 1/2 ripe avocado
- 1 large egg
- Salt and pepper to taste
- Fresh parsley (optional)

DIRECTIONS

1. Mash avocado on toasted gluten-free bread.
2. Bring a pot of water to a simmer, crack egg into a bowl.
3. Create a whirlpool in water and gently add the egg.
4. Poach for 3-4 minutes until whites are set.
5. Place poached egg on avocado toast, season with salt, pepper, and parsley.
6. Serve immediately.

NUTRITIONAL INFO

- Calories: 250
- Protein: 8g
- Fat: 16g
- Carbs: 20g

FRUIT AND COTTAGE CHEESE BOWL

(Serves 1 | 5 mins)

INGREDIENTS

- 1/2 cup lactose-free cottage cheese
- 1/4 cup pineapple chunks (fresh or canned in juice)
- 1 tbsp walnuts (chopped)
- 1 tsp maple syrup (optional)

DIRECTIONS

1. Scoop cottage cheese into a bowl.
2. Top with pineapple chunks.
3. Sprinkle with chopped walnuts.
4. Drizzle with maple syrup, if desired.
5. Serve immediately.

NUTRITIONAL INFO

- Calories: 200
- Protein: 12g
- Fat: 8g
- Carbs: 20g

ALMOND FLOUR PANCAKES

(Serves 2 | 15 mins)

INGREDIENTS

- 1/2 cup almond flour
- 1 large egg
- 1/4 cup lactose-free milk
- 1/4 tsp baking powder
- 1/2 tsp vanilla extract
- 1 tsp olive oil for cooking

DIRECTIONS

1. Mix almond flour, egg, milk, baking powder, and vanilla until smooth.
2. Heat oil in a non-stick pan over medium heat.
3. Pour small amounts of batter to form pancakes.
4. Cook until bubbles form on top, flip, and cook until golden.
5. Serve with fresh berries or maple syrup.

NUTRITIONAL INFO

- Calories: 150
- Protein: 6g
- Fat: 10g
- Carbs: 6g

ALMOND FLOUR PANCAKES

(Serves 2 | 15 mins)

INGREDIENTS

- 1/2 cup almond flour
- 1 large egg
- 1/4 cup lactose-free milk
- 1/4 tsp baking powder
- 1/2 tsp vanilla extract
- 1 tsp olive oil for cooking

DIRECTIONS

1. Mix almond flour, egg, milk, baking powder, and vanilla until smooth.
2. Heat oil in a non-stick pan over medium heat.
3. Pour small amounts of batter to form pancakes.
4. Cook until bubbles form on top, flip, and cook until golden.
5. Serve with fresh berries or maple syrup.

NUTRITIONAL INFO

- Calories: 150
- Protein: 6g
- Fat: 10g
- Carbs: 6g

QUINOA BREAKFAST PORRIDGE

(Serves 2 | 15 mins)

INGREDIENTS

- 1/2 cup cooked quinoa
- 1 cup lactose-free milk
- 1 tsp cinnamon
- 1 tbsp maple syrup
- 1/4 cup raspberries

DIRECTIONS

1. In a pot, combine quinoa, milk, and cinnamon.
2. Heat over medium heat, stirring occasionally, until warm.
3. Stir in maple syrup.
4. Serve topped with raspberries.

NUTRITIONAL INFO

- Calories: 180
- Protein: 6g
- Fat: 3g
- Carbs: 30g

EGG AND BELL PEPPER CUPS

(Serves 2 | 20 mins)

INGREDIENTS

- 2 bell peppers (halved, seeds removed)
- 4 large eggs
- Salt and pepper to taste
- Fresh parsley (for garnish)

DIRECTIONS

1. Preheat oven to 375°F (190°C).
2. Place bell pepper halves on a baking tray.
3. Crack an egg into each bell pepper half.
4. Season with salt and pepper.
5. Bake for 15-20 minutes, or until eggs are cooked.
6. Garnish with parsley and serve.

NUTRITIONAL INFO

- Calories: 120
- Protein: 8g
- Fat: 7g
- Carbs: 6g

BUCKWHEAT PORRIDGE WITH STRAWBERRIES

(Serves 1 | 10 mins)

INGREDIENTS

- 1/4 cup buckwheat groats
- 1 cup water
- 1/4 cup strawberries (sliced)
- 1 tsp maple syrup

DIRECTIONS

1. Rinse buckwheat groats and add to a pot with water.
2. Bring to a boil, then simmer for 8-10 minutes.
3. Serve porridge with strawberries on top.
4. Drizzle with maple syrup before serving.

NUTRITIONAL INFO

- Calories: 150
- Protein: 4g
- Fat: 1g
- Carbs: 30g

BERRY CHIA PUDDING

(Serves 2 | 5 mins prep + 4 hrs chilling)

INGREDIENTS

- 1 cup lactose-free milk
- 3 tbsp chia seeds
- 1/4 cup mixed berries (blueberries, raspberries)
- 1 tbsp maple syrup

DIRECTIONS

1. In a bowl, combine milk, chia seeds, and maple syrup.
2. Stir well, let sit for 5 minutes.
3. Stir again to prevent clumping.
4. Cover and refrigerate for at least 4 hours.
5. Top with mixed berries before serving.

NUTRITIONAL INFO

- Calories: 180
- Protein: 4g
- Fat: 8g
- Carbs: 22g

SPINACH AND FETA BREAKFAST WRAP

(Serves 1 | 10 mins)

INGREDIENTS

- 1 gluten-free tortilla
- 1/2 cup fresh spinach
- 1/4 cup crumbled feta cheese (lactose-free)
- 1 large egg
- 1 tsp olive oil

DIRECTIONS

1. Heat oil in a pan, sauté spinach until wilted.
2. Whisk egg, scramble in pan, and mix with spinach.
3. Place scrambled mixture on tortilla.
4. Top with feta cheese.
5. Fold tortilla and serve.

NUTRITIONAL INFO

- Calories: 250
- Protein: 12g
- Fat: 14g
- Carbs: 20g

MAPLE-CINNAMON RICE PORRIDGE

(Serves 2 | 10 mins)

INGREDIENTS

- 1 cup cooked rice (white or brown)
- 1 cup lactose-free milk
- 1 tbsp maple syrup
- 1/2 tsp ground cinnamon

DIRECTIONS

1. Combine rice and milk in a pot over medium heat.
2. Stir in maple syrup and cinnamon.
3. Heat until warm, stirring occasionally.
4. Serve in bowls.

NUTRITIONAL INFO
- Calories: 180
- Protein: 5g
- Fat: 2g
- Carbs: 36g

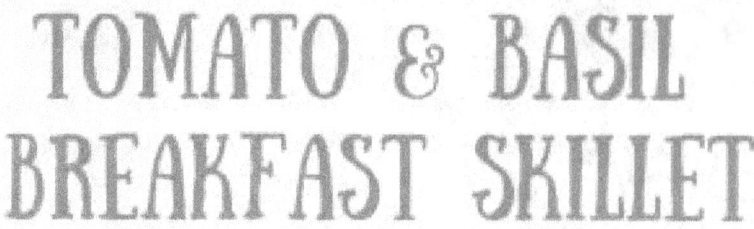

TOMATO & BASIL BREAKFAST SKILLET

(Serves 2 | 15 mins)

INGREDIENTS

- 2 large eggs
- 1 cup cherry tomatoes (halved)
- 1/4 cup fresh basil leaves
- 1 tbsp olive oil
- Salt and pepper to taste

DIRECTIONS

1. Heat olive oil in a skillet over medium heat.
2. Add cherry tomatoes, sauté until softened.
3. Make two wells in tomatoes, crack an egg into each.
4. Cover skillet and cook eggs until whites are set.
5. Season with salt, pepper, and fresh basil.
6. Serve immediately.

NUTRITIONAL INFO

- Calories: 150
- Protein: 6g
- Fat: 11g
- Carbs: 5g

Fish And Seafood Recipes

LEMON HERB GRILLED SALMON

(Serves 2 | 15 mins)

INGREDIENTS

- 2 salmon fillets
- 1 tbsp olive oil
- Juice of 1 lemon
- 1 tbsp fresh parsley (chopped)
- Salt and pepper to taste

DIRECTIONS

1. Mix olive oil, lemon juice, parsley, salt, and pepper.
2. Coat salmon fillets with the marinade.
3. Heat a grill or pan over medium heat.
4. Grill salmon for 4-5 mins on each side until cooked through.
5. Serve warm with an additional squeeze of lemon.

NUTRITIONAL INFO

- Calories: 250
- Protein: 23g
- Fat: 16g
- Carbs: 2g

GARLIC-INFUSED SHRIMP STIR-FRY

(Serves 2 | 10 mins)

INGREDIENTS

- 200g shrimp (peeled and deveined)
- 1 tbsp garlic-infused olive oil
- 1 cup bell peppers (sliced)
- 1 cup zucchini (sliced)
- 1 tbsp soy sauce

DIRECTIONS

1. Heat garlic-infused oil in a pan over medium heat.
2. Add shrimp and cook until pink, then set aside.
3. Stir-fry bell peppers and zucchini until tender.
4. Return shrimp to pan and add soy sauce.
5. Stir well and cook for another 1-2 mins.
6. Serve immediately.

NUTRITIONAL INFO

- Calories: 150
- Protein: 25g
- Fat: 6g
- Carbs: 5g

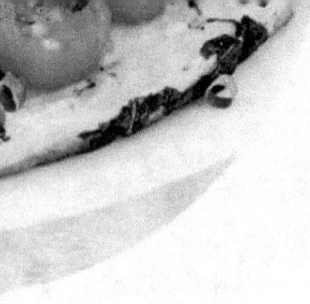

BAKED COD WITH DILL AND LEMON
(Serves 2 | 20 mins)

INGREDIENTS

- 2 cod fillets
- 1 tbsp olive oil
- Juice of 1/2 lemon
- 1 tbsp fresh dill (chopped)
- Salt and pepper to taste

DIRECTIONS

1. Preheat oven to 375°F (190°C).
2. Place cod fillets in a baking dish.
3. Drizzle with olive oil, lemon juice, dill, salt, and pepper.
4. Bake for 15-20 mins until fish is opaque and flakes easily.
5. Serve with additional fresh dill.

NUTRITIONAL INFO

- Calories: 120
- Protein: 25g
- Fat: 3g
- Carbs: 0g

PAN-SEARED SCALLOPS WITH LIME

(Serves 2 | 10 mins)

INGREDIENTS

- 8-10 large scallops
- 1 tbsp olive oil
- Juice of 1 lime
- Fresh cilantro (chopped)
- Salt and pepper to taste

DIRECTIONS

1. Heat olive oil in a pan over medium-high heat.
2. Season scallops with salt and pepper.
3. Sear scallops for 2 mins on each side until golden.
4. Remove from heat and drizzle with lime juice.
5. Garnish with fresh cilantro.

NUTRITIONAL INFO

- Calories: 130
- Protein: 22g
- Fat: 4g
- Carbs: 3g

CILANTRO LIME SHRIMP SKEWERS

(Serves 2 | 15 mins)

INGREDIENTS

- 200g shrimp (peeled and deveined)
- Juice of 1 lime
- 1 tbsp olive oil
- Fresh cilantro (chopped)
- Salt to taste

DIRECTIONS

1. Mix lime juice, olive oil, cilantro, and salt.
2. Marinate shrimp for 10 mins.
3. Thread shrimp onto skewers.
4. Grill or pan-cook for 2-3 mins per side until pink.
5. Serve immediately.

NUTRITIONAL INFO

- Calories: 120
- Protein: 20g
- Fat: 5g
- Carbs: 2g

SESAME-CRUSTED TUNA STEAKS

(Serves 2 | 10 mins)

INGREDIENTS

- 2 tuna steaks
- 2 tbsp sesame seeds
- 1 tbsp olive oil
- 1 tsp soy sauce
- Salt and pepper to taste

DIRECTIONS

1. Season tuna with soy sauce, salt, and pepper.
2. Press sesame seeds onto both sides of tuna.
3. Heat olive oil in a pan over medium-high heat.
4. Sear tuna for 1-2 mins per side (until desired doneness).
5. Serve immediately.

NUTRITIONAL INFO

- Calories: 220
- Protein: 24g
- Fat: 12g
- Carbs: 1g

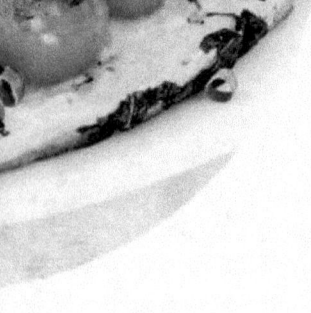

BAKED TILAPIA WITH PAPRIKA AND LEMON

(Serves 2 | 15 mins)

INGREDIENTS

- 2 tilapia fillets
- 1 tbsp olive oil
- 1/2 tsp paprika
- Juice of 1/2 lemon
- Salt and pepper to taste

DIRECTIONS

1. Preheat oven to 375°F (190°C).
2. Place tilapia in a baking dish, drizzle with olive oil.
3. Season with paprika, lemon juice, salt, and pepper.
4. Bake for 12-15 mins until fish flakes easily.
5. Serve warm.

NUTRITIONAL INFO

- Calories: 110
- Protein: 22g
- Fat: 3g
- Carbs: 1g

GARLIC-INFUSED MACKEREL WITH HERBS

(Serves 2 | 20 mins)

INGREDIENTS

- 2 mackerel fillets
- 1 tbsp garlic-infused olive oil
- 1 tbsp fresh rosemary (chopped)
- Salt and pepper to taste
- Juice of 1/2 lemon

DIRECTIONS

1. Preheat oven to 375°F (190°C).
2. Place mackerel on a baking sheet, brush with oil.
3. Season with rosemary, salt, and pepper.
4. Bake for 15-20 mins until cooked through.
5. Squeeze lemon juice over before serving.

NUTRITIONAL INFO

- Calories: 200
- Protein: 24g
- Fat: 10g
- Carbs: 1g

LEMON-GINGER BAKED TROUT

(Serves 2 | 20 mins)

INGREDIENTS

- 2 trout fillets
- 1 tbsp olive oil
- 1 tsp fresh ginger (grated)
- Juice of 1 lemon
- Salt and pepper to taste

DIRECTIONS

1. Preheat oven to 375°F (190°C).
2. Mix olive oil, ginger, lemon juice, salt, and pepper.
3. Place trout on a baking sheet, drizzle with mixture.
4. Bake for 15-20 mins until flaky and cooked through.
5. Serve warm with lemon slices.

NUTRITIONAL INFO

- Calories: 180
- Protein: 20g
- Fat: 9g
- Carbs: 1g

HERB-CRUSTED BAKED HADDOCK

(Serves 2 | 20 mins)

INGREDIENTS

- 2 haddock fillets
- 2 tbsp gluten-free breadcrumbs
- 1 tbsp fresh parsley (chopped)
- 1 tbsp olive oil
- Salt and pepper to taste

DIRECTIONS

1. Preheat oven to 375°F (190°C).
2. Mix breadcrumbs, parsley, salt, and pepper.
3. Brush haddock with olive oil and coat with breadcrumb mixture.
4. Place on a baking sheet and bake for 15-20 mins until golden.
5. Serve with a side of greens.

NUTRITIONAL INFO

- Calories: 170
- Protein: 22g
- Fat: 6g
- Carbs: 8g

BASIL LEMON GRILLED SWORDFISH

(Serves 2 | 15 mins)

INGREDIENTS

- 2 swordfish steaks
- 1 tbsp olive oil
- Juice of 1 lemon
- Fresh basil leaves (chopped)
- Salt and pepper to taste

DIRECTIONS

1. Mix olive oil, lemon juice, basil, salt, and pepper.
2. Marinate swordfish steaks for 10 minutes.
3. Heat grill or pan over medium heat.
4. Cook steaks for 3-4 mins on each side until done.
5. Serve with extra lemon juice.

NUTRITIONAL INFO

- Calories: 220
- Protein: 25g
- Fat: 12g
- Carbs: 1g

CRISPY BAKED SOLE FILLETS

(Serves 2 | 15 mins)

INGREDIENTS

- 2 sole fillets
- 2 tbsp gluten-free breadcrumbs
- 1 tbsp olive oil
- 1/2 tsp paprika
- Salt and pepper to taste

DIRECTIONS

1. Preheat oven to 375°F (190°C).
2. Mix breadcrumbs, paprika, salt, and pepper.
3. Brush fillets with olive oil, coat with breadcrumb mixture.
4. Place on a baking sheet and bake for 10-12 mins until crispy.
5. Serve immediately.

NUTRITIONAL INFO

- Calories: 150
- Protein: 22g
- Fat: 5g
- Carbs: 6g

GINGER SOY SHRIMP SAUTÉ

(Serves 2 | 10 mins)

INGREDIENTS

- 200g shrimp (peeled and deveined)
- 1 tbsp ginger (grated)
- 1 tbsp soy sauce
- 1 tbsp sesame oil
- 1 tbsp green onion tops (chopped)

DIRECTIONS

1. Heat sesame oil in a pan over medium heat.
2. Add ginger and sauté until fragrant.
3. Add shrimp and soy sauce; cook until shrimp turns pink.
4. Sprinkle green onion tops before serving.
5. Serve with rice or steamed vegetables.

NUTRITIONAL INFO

- Calories: 130
- Protein: 23g
- Fat: 4g
- Carbs: 2g

LEMON DILL POACHED HADDOCK

(Serves 2 | 15 mins)

INGREDIENTS

- 2 haddock fillets
- 2 cups water
- Juice of 1 lemon
- 1 tbsp fresh dill (chopped)
- Salt and pepper to taste

DIRECTIONS

1. Bring water, lemon juice, salt, and pepper to a simmer.
2. Add haddock fillets and poach for 8-10 mins.
3. Remove fillets and let drain.
4. Garnish with fresh dill before serving.
5. Serve warm.

NUTRITIONAL INFO

- Calories: 100
- Protein: 21g
- Fat: 1g
- Carbs: 1g

BAKED MAHI-MAHI WITH FRESH HERBS

(Serves 2 | 15 mins)

INGREDIENTS

- 2 mahi-mahi fillets
- 1 tbsp olive oil
- 1 tbsp fresh thyme (chopped)
- 1 tbsp fresh rosemary (chopped)
- Salt and pepper to taste

DIRECTIONS

1. Preheat oven to 375°F (190°C).
2. Brush fillets with olive oil, season with thyme, rosemary, salt, and pepper.
3. Place on a baking dish and bake for 12-15 mins.
4. Serve immediately.

NUTRITIONAL INFO

- Calories: 180
- Protein: 24g
- Fat: 8g
- Carbs: 0g

PAPRIKA GRILLED PRAWNS

(Serves 2 | 10 mins)

INGREDIENTS

- 200g prawns (peeled and deveined)
- 1 tbsp olive oil
- 1/2 tsp paprika
- 1 tbsp lemon juice
- Salt to taste

DIRECTIONS

1. Toss prawns with olive oil, paprika, lemon juice, and salt.
2. Thread prawns onto skewers.
3. Grill over medium heat for 2-3 mins per side.
4. Serve warm with extra lemon juice.

NUTRITIONAL INFO

- Calories: 120
- Protein: 22g
- Fat: 5g
- Carbs: 1g

SESAME-CRUSTED SALMON

(Serves 2 | 15 mins)

INGREDIENTS

- 2 salmon fillets
- 2 tbsp sesame seeds
- 1 tbsp olive oil
- Salt and pepper to taste

DIRECTIONS

1. Season salmon with salt and pepper.
2. Coat salmon with sesame seeds.
3. Heat olive oil in a pan over medium heat.
4. Cook salmon for 3-4 mins on each side until crispy.
5. Serve with a side of steamed greens.

NUTRITIONAL INFO

- Calories: 240
- Protein: 22g
- Fat: 14g
- Carbs: 2g

LIME AND CILANTRO GRILLED TILAPIA

(Serves 2 | 10 mins)

INGREDIENTS

- 2 tilapia fillets
- Juice of 1 lime
- 1 tbsp olive oil
- Fresh cilantro (chopped)
- Salt to taste

DIRECTIONS

1. Mix lime juice, olive oil, cilantro, and salt.
2. Marinate tilapia fillets for 10 mins.
3. Grill for 3-4 mins per side until cooked.
4. Serve with extra lime juice and cilantro.

NUTRITIONAL INFO

- Calories: 110
- Protein: 22g
- Fat: 4g
- Carbs: 1g

HERB-ROASTED SEA BASS

(Serves 2 | 20 mins)

INGREDIENTS

- 2 sea bass fillets
- 1 tbsp olive oil
- 1 tbsp fresh parsley (chopped)
- 1/2 tsp dried thyme
- Salt and pepper to taste

DIRECTIONS

1. Preheat oven to 375°F (190°C).
2. Rub sea bass with olive oil, parsley, thyme, salt, and pepper.
3. Place on a baking tray and bake for 15-20 mins.
4. Serve warm with a lemon wedge.

NUTRITIONAL INFO

- Calories: 180
- Protein: 25g
- Fat: 7g
- Carbs: 0g

CUMIN-SPICED GRILLED HALIBUT

(Serves 2 | 15 mins)

INGREDIENTS

- 2 halibut fillets
- 1 tbsp olive oil
- 1/2 tsp cumin powder
- Salt and pepper to taste
- Fresh lemon juice (for serving)

DIRECTIONS

1. Rub halibut with olive oil, cumin, salt, and pepper.
2. Heat grill or pan over medium heat.
3. Cook fillets for 4-5 mins on each side until flaky.
4. Squeeze lemon juice over before serving.

NUTRITIONAL INFO

- Calories: 200
- Protein: 26g
- Fat: 9g
- Carbs: 0g

CHILI LIME GRILLED TUNA

(Serves 2 | 10 mins)

INGREDIENTS

- 2 tuna steaks
- Juice of 1 lime
- 1/2 tsp chili powder
- 1 tbsp olive oil
- Salt to taste

DIRECTIONS

1. Mix lime juice, chili powder, olive oil, and salt.
2. Marinate tuna steaks for 5 minutes.
3. Grill or pan-sear steaks for 2-3 mins per side.
4. Serve with extra lime juice.

NUTRITIONAL INFO

- Calories: 220
- Protein: 25g
- Fat: 11g
- Carbs: 1g

Poultry Recipes

LEMON HERB GRILLED CHICKEN BREAST

(Serves 2 | 15 mins)

INGREDIENTS

- 2 chicken breasts
- 1 tbsp olive oil
- Juice of 1 lemon
- 1 tbsp fresh parsley (chopped)
- Salt and pepper to taste

DIRECTIONS

1. Mix olive oil, lemon juice, parsley, salt, and pepper.
2. Marinate chicken breasts for 10 minutes.
3. Heat a grill or pan over medium heat.
4. Grill chicken for 5-6 mins per side until cooked through.
5. Serve with fresh parsley.

NUTRITIONAL INFO

- Calories: 180
- Protein: 30g
- Fat: 7g
- Carbs: 1g

ROSEMARY BAKED CHICKEN THIGHS

(Serves 2 | 15 mins)

INGREDIENTS

- 4 chicken thighs (skinless, bone-in)
- 1 tbsp olive oil
- 1 tsp dried rosemary
- Salt and pepper to taste
- Juice of 1/2 lemon

DIRECTIONS

1. Preheat oven to 375°F (190°C).
2. Rub chicken thighs with olive oil, rosemary, salt, and pepper.
3. Place in a baking dish, drizzle with lemon juice.
4. Bake for 20-25 mins until cooked through.
5. Serve warm.

NUTRITIONAL INFO

- Calories: 200
- Protein: 25g
- Fat: 12g
- Carbs: 1g

GARLIC-INFUSED CHICKEN STIR-FRY

(Serves 2 | 15 mins)

INGREDIENTS

- 2 chicken breasts (sliced)
- 1 tbsp garlic-infused olive oil
- 1 cup bell peppers (sliced)
- 1 cup zucchini (sliced)
- 1 tbsp soy sauce

DIRECTIONS

1. Heat garlic-infused oil in a pan over medium heat.
2. Add chicken and cook until browned.
3. Add bell peppers and zucchini; stir-fry until tender.
4. Stir in soy sauce and cook for another 2 mins.
5. Serve immediately.

NUTRITIONAL INFO

- Calories: 180
- Protein: 28g
- Fat: 6g
- Carbs: 4g

BASIL LIME CHICKEN SKEWERS

(Serves 2 | 15 mins)

INGREDIENTS

- 2 chicken breasts (cubed)
- Juice of 1 lime
- 1 tbsp olive oil
- Fresh basil (chopped)
- Salt to taste

DIRECTIONS

1. Mix lime juice, olive oil, basil, and salt.
2. Marinate chicken cubes for 10 mins.
3. Thread chicken onto skewers.
4. Grill for 3-4 mins per side until cooked.
5. Serve warm.

NUTRITIONAL INFO

- Calories: 170
- Protein: 29g
- Fat: 5g
- Carbs: 1g

PAPRIKA BAKED TURKEY BREAST

(Serves 2 | 25 mins)

INGREDIENTS

- 2 turkey breast cutlets
- 1 tbsp olive oil
- 1/2 tsp paprika
- Salt and pepper to taste
- Fresh parsley for garnish

DIRECTIONS

1. Preheat oven to 375°F (190°C).
2. Rub turkey with olive oil, paprika, salt, and pepper.
3. Place on a baking sheet and bake for 20-25 mins.
4. Garnish with parsley before serving.
5. Serve warm.

NUTRITIONAL INFO

- Calories: 160
- Protein: 28g
- Fat: 5g
- Carbs: 1g

GINGER LIME TURKEY MEATBALLS

(Serves 3 | 20 mins)

INGREDIENTS

- 300g ground turkey
- 1 tbsp ginger (grated)
- Juice of 1 lime
- 1 tbsp fresh cilantro (chopped)
- Salt to taste

DIRECTIONS

1. Mix turkey, ginger, lime juice, cilantro, and salt.
2. Form into small meatballs.
3. Heat a non-stick pan over medium heat.
4. Cook meatballs for 5-6 mins per side until browned.
5. Serve warm.

NUTRITIONAL INFO

- Calories: 140
- Protein: 24g
- Fat: 4g
- Carbs: 1g

BALSAMIC GLAZED CHICKEN DRUMSTICKS

(Serves 2 | 25 mins)

INGREDIENTS

- 4 chicken drumsticks
- 2 tbsp balsamic vinegar
- 1 tbsp olive oil
- 1 tsp dried thyme
- Salt and pepper to taste

DIRECTIONS

1. Mix balsamic vinegar, olive oil, thyme, salt, and pepper.
2. Coat drumsticks with the mixture.
3. Preheat oven to 375°F (190°C).
4. Bake for 20-25 mins until cooked through.
5. Serve with extra balsamic glaze.

NUTRITIONAL INFO

- Calories: 180
- Protein: 22g
- Fat: 9g
- Carbs: 3g

TURMERIC LEMON ROASTED CHICKEN WINGS

(Serves 2 | 25 mins)

INGREDIENTS

- 6 chicken wings
- 1 tbsp olive oil
- 1 tsp ground turmeric
- Juice of 1/2 lemon
- Salt and pepper to taste

DIRECTIONS

1. Mix olive oil, turmeric, lemon juice, salt, and pepper.
2. Coat chicken wings with the mixture.
3. Preheat oven to 400°F (200°C).
4. Roast for 20-25 mins until golden and cooked.
5. Serve warm.

NUTRITIONAL INFO

- Calories: 210
- Protein: 18g
- Fat: 15g
- Carbs: 1g

GRILLED JERK-SPICED CHICKEN THIGHS

(Serves 2 | 20 mins)

INGREDIENTS

- 4 chicken thighs (skinless)
- 1 tbsp olive oil
- 1 tsp jerk seasoning (low FODMAP blend)
- Salt to taste
- Juice of 1/2 lime

DIRECTIONS

1. Mix olive oil, jerk seasoning, lime juice, and salt.
2. Coat chicken thighs with the mixture.
3. Heat grill over medium heat.
4. Grill for 6-7 mins per side until cooked through.
5. Serve immediately.

NUTRITIONAL INFO

- Calories: 220
- Protein: 26g
- Fat: 12g
- Carbs: 2g

CUMIN SPICED GRILLED TURKEY BREAST

(Serves 2 | 15 mins)

INGREDIENTS

- 2 turkey breast cutlets
- 1 tbsp olive oil
- 1/2 tsp ground cumin
- Salt and pepper to taste
- Fresh cilantro for garnish

DIRECTIONS

1. Mix olive oil, cumin, salt, and pepper.
2. Rub the mixture over turkey cutlets.
3. Heat grill over medium heat.
4. Grill for 5-6 mins per side until done.
5. Garnish with cilantro before serving.

NUTRITIONAL INFO

- Calories: 150
- Protein: 30g
- Fat: 4g
- Carbs: 1g

MAPLE MUSTARD CHICKEN BREASTS

(Serves 2 | 20 mins)

INGREDIENTS

- 2 chicken breasts
- 1 tbsp maple syrup
- 1 tbsp Dijon mustard
- 1 tbsp olive oil
- Salt and pepper to taste

DIRECTIONS

1. Mix maple syrup, mustard, olive oil, salt, and pepper.
2. Marinate chicken breasts for 10 minutes.
3. Heat a pan over medium heat.
4. Cook chicken for 6-7 mins per side until golden and cooked.
5. Serve warm with sauce drizzled over.

NUTRITIONAL INFO

- Calories: 200
- Protein: 30g
- Fat: 6g
- Carbs: 4g

CITRUS GRILLED CHICKEN THIGHS

(Serves 2 | 15 mins)

INGREDIENTS

- 4 chicken thighs (skinless)
- Juice of 1 orange
- 1 tbsp olive oil
- Salt and pepper to taste
- Fresh thyme for garnish

DIRECTIONS

1. Mix orange juice, olive oil, salt, and pepper.
2. Marinate chicken thighs for 10 mins.
3. Grill over medium heat for 5-6 mins per side.
4. Serve garnished with fresh thyme.

NUTRITIONAL INFO

- Calories: 180
- Protein: 24g
- Fat: 8g
- Carbs: 2g

ROSEMARY LEMON TURKEY BURGERS

(Serves 3 | 15 mins)

INGREDIENTS

- 300g ground turkey
- 1 tbsp fresh rosemary (chopped)
- Juice of 1/2 lemon
- 1 tbsp olive oil
- Salt and pepper to taste

DIRECTIONS

1. Mix ground turkey, rosemary, lemon juice, salt, and pepper.
2. Form into 3 patties.
3. Heat oil in a pan over medium heat.
4. Cook patties for 5-6 mins per side until browned.
5. Serve on a gluten-free bun or lettuce wrap.

NUTRITIONAL INFO

- Calories: 150
- Protein: 22g
- Fat: 6g
- Carbs: 1g

THYME ROASTED CHICKEN DRUMSTICKS

(Serves 2 | 25 mins)

INGREDIENTS

- 4 chicken drumsticks
- 1 tbsp olive oil
- 1 tsp dried thyme
- Salt and pepper to taste
- Juice of 1/2 lemon

DIRECTIONS

1. Preheat oven to 375°F (190°C).
2. Rub drumsticks with olive oil, thyme, salt, and pepper.
3. Roast for 20-25 mins until golden and cooked.
4. Drizzle with lemon juice before serving.

NUTRITIONAL INFO

- Calories: 170
- Protein: 22g
- Fat: 9g
- Carbs: 1g

BASIL PESTO BAKED CHICKEN

(Serves 2 | 20 mins)

INGREDIENTS

- 2 chicken breasts
- 2 tbsp basil pesto (Low FODMAP brand)
- 1 tbsp olive oil
- Salt to taste
- Fresh basil for garnish

DIRECTIONS

1. Preheat oven to 375°F (190°C).
2. Rub chicken with pesto, olive oil, and salt.
3. Place in a baking dish and bake for 15-20 mins.
4. Garnish with fresh basil before serving.

NUTRITIONAL INFO

- Calories: 210
- Protein: 30g
- Fat: 8g
- Carbs: 2g

HONEY LIME GRILLED TURKEY CUTLETS

(Serves 2 | 15 mins)

INGREDIENTS

- 2 turkey cutlets
- 1 tbsp honey
- Juice of 1 lime
- 1 tbsp olive oil
- Salt to taste

DIRECTIONS

1. Mix honey, lime juice, olive oil, and salt.
2. Marinate turkey cutlets for 10 mins.
3. Grill over medium heat for 4-5 mins per side.
4. Serve immediately with extra lime juice.

NUTRITIONAL INFO

- Calories: 170
- Protein: 25g
- Fat: 5g
- Carbs: 3g

SAGE BAKED CHICKEN BREASTS

(Serves 2 | 20 mins)

INGREDIENTS

- 2 chicken breasts
- 1 tbsp olive oil
- 1 tsp dried sage
- Salt and pepper to taste
- Fresh parsley for garnish

DIRECTIONS

1. Preheat oven to 375°F (190°C).
2. Rub chicken with olive oil, sage, salt, and pepper.
3. Place in a baking dish and bake for 15-20 mins.
4. Garnish with parsley before serving.

NUTRITIONAL INFO

- Calories: 180
- Protein: 30g
- Fat: 6g
- Carbs: 1g

TERIYAKI TURKEY STIR-FRY

(Serves 2 | 15 mins)

INGREDIENTS

- 200g turkey breast (sliced)
- 1 tbsp soy sauce
- 1 tbsp maple syrup
- 1 cup broccoli florets
- 1 tbsp sesame oil

DIRECTIONS

1. Heat sesame oil in a pan over medium heat.
2. Add turkey and cook until browned.
3. Add broccoli and stir-fry for 2-3 mins.
4. Stir in soy sauce and maple syrup; cook for 1 min.
5. Serve immediately.

NUTRITIONAL INFO

- Calories: 160
- Protein: 25g
- Fat: 5g
- Carbs: 4g

OREGANO LEMON CHICKEN THIGHS

(Serves 2 | 20 mins)

INGREDIENTS

- 4 chicken thighs (skinless)
- 1 tbsp olive oil
- 1 tsp dried oregano
- Juice of 1 lemon
- Salt to taste

DIRECTIONS

1. Preheat oven to 375°F (190°C).
2. Mix olive oil, oregano, lemon juice, and salt.
3. Rub mixture over chicken thighs.
4. Bake for 20 mins until golden and cooked.
5. Serve warm.

NUTRITIONAL INFO

- Calories: 200
- Protein: 26g
- Fat: 10g
- Carbs: 1g

CUMIN LIME GRILLED CHICKEN

(Serves 2 | 15 mins)

INGREDIENTS

- 2 chicken breasts
- 1 tbsp olive oil
- 1/2 tsp ground cumin
- Juice of 1 lime
- Salt to taste

DIRECTIONS

1. Mix olive oil, cumin, lime juice, and salt.
2. Marinate chicken breasts for 10 mins.
3. Grill over medium heat for 5-6 mins per side.
4. Serve immediately.

NUTRITIONAL INFO

- Calories: 190
- Protein: 30g
- Fat: 7g
- Carbs: 1g

CILANTRO LIME TURKEY MEATBALLS

(Serves 3 | 20 mins)

INGREDIENTS

- 300g ground turkey
- 1 tbsp fresh cilantro (chopped)
- Juice of 1 lime
- 1 tbsp olive oil
- Salt and pepper to taste

DIRECTIONS

1. Mix turkey, cilantro, lime juice, salt, and pepper.
2. Form into small meatballs.
3. Heat oil in a pan over medium heat.
4. Cook meatballs for 5-6 mins per side until browned.
5. Serve warm with extra cilantro.

NUTRITIONAL INFO

- Calories: 150
- Protein: 24g
- Fat: 6g
- Carbs: 1g

Vegetable And Salad Recipes

ROASTED CARROT AND ZUCCHINI SALAD

(Serves 2 | 20 mins)

INGREDIENTS

- 2 carrots (sliced)
- 1 zucchini (sliced)
- 1 tbsp olive oil
- 1 tbsp fresh parsley (chopped)
- Salt and pepper to taste

DIRECTIONS

1. Preheat oven to 400°F (200°C).
2. Toss carrots and zucchini with olive oil, salt, and pepper.
3. Roast for 15-20 mins until tender.
4. Remove and let cool slightly.
5. Mix with fresh parsley and serve.

NUTRITIONAL INFO

- Calories: 80
- Carbs: 10g
- Fat: 4g
- Fiber: 3g

SPINACH AND STRAWBERRY SALAD

(Serves 2 | 5 mins)

INGREDIENTS

- 2 cups baby spinach
- 1/2 cup strawberries (sliced)
- 1 tbsp balsamic vinegar
- 1 tbsp olive oil
- Salt and pepper to taste

DIRECTIONS

1. Place spinach and strawberries in a bowl.
2. Mix balsamic vinegar, olive oil, salt, and pepper.
3. Drizzle dressing over salad.
4. Toss gently and serve.

NUTRITIONAL INFO

- Calories: 70
- Carbs: 8g
- Fat: 4g
- Fiber: 2g

CUCUMBER DILL SALAD

(Serves 2 | 10 mins)

INGREDIENTS

- 1 cucumber (sliced)
- 1 tbsp fresh dill (chopped)
- 1 tbsp lemon juice
- 1 tbsp olive oil
- Salt to taste

DIRECTIONS

1. Place cucumber slices in a bowl.
2. Mix dill, lemon juice, olive oil, and salt.
3. Drizzle dressing over cucumbers.
4. Toss to combine and serve chilled.

NUTRITIONAL INFO

- Calories: 40
- Carbs: 4g
- Fat: 3g
- Fiber: 1g

ROASTED BELL PEPPERS AND EGGPLANT

(Serves 2 | 25 mins)

INGREDIENTS

- 1 red bell pepper (sliced)
- 1 yellow bell pepper (sliced)
- 1 small eggplant (cubed)
- 2 tbsp olive oil
- Salt and pepper to taste

DIRECTIONS

1. Preheat oven to 400°F (200°C).
2. Toss bell peppers and eggplant with olive oil, salt, and pepper.
3. Spread on a baking sheet.
4. Roast for 20-25 mins until tender.
5. Serve warm or chilled.

NUTRITIONAL INFO

- Calories: 90
- Carbs: 10g
- Fat: 5g
- Fiber: 3g

SIMPLE TOMATO AND BASIL SALAD

(Serves 2 | 25 mins)

INGREDIENTS

- 2 medium tomatoes (sliced)
- Fresh basil leaves
- 1 tbsp olive oil
- 1 tsp balsamic vinegar
- Salt and pepper to taste

DIRECTIONS

1. Layer tomato slices on a plate.
2. Top with basil leaves.
3. Drizzle with olive oil and balsamic vinegar.
4. Sprinkle with salt and pepper before serving.

NUTRITIONAL INFO

- Calories: 50
- Carbs: 6g
- Fat: 3g
- Fiber: 2g

ROASTED GREEN BEANS WITH LEMON ZEST

(Serves 2 | 15 mins)

INGREDIENTS

- 2 cups green beans (trimmed)
- 1 tbsp olive oil
- Zest of 1 lemon
- Salt and pepper to taste

DIRECTIONS

1. Preheat oven to 400°F (200°C).
2. Toss green beans with olive oil, salt, and pepper.
3. Roast for 12-15 mins until tender.
4. Sprinkle with lemon zest before serving.

NUTRITIONAL INFO

- Calories: 60
- Carbs: 7g
- Fat: 4g
- Fiber: 3g

GRILLED ASPARAGUS WITH SEA SALT

(Serves 2 | 10 mins)

INGREDIENTS

- 1 bunch asparagus (trimmed)
- 1 tbsp olive oil
- Sea salt to taste
- Fresh lemon juice

DIRECTIONS

1. Heat a grill or pan over medium heat.
2. Toss asparagus with olive oil and sea salt.
3. Grill for 5-6 mins, turning occasionally.
4. Drizzle with lemon juice before serving.

NUTRITIONAL INFO

- Calories: 45
- Carbs: 4g
- Fat: 3g
- Fiber: 2g

CARROT AND PARSNIP MASH

(Serves 2 | 15 mins)

INGREDIENTS

- 2 carrots (peeled, chopped)
- 2 parsnips (peeled, chopped)
- 1 tbsp olive oil
- Salt and pepper to taste
- Fresh parsley (chopped)

DIRECTIONS

1. Boil carrots and parsnips until soft (about 10 mins).
2. Drain and mash with olive oil, salt, and pepper.
3. Top with fresh parsley.
4. Serve warm.

NUTRITIONAL INFO

- Calories: 80
- Carbs: 15g
- Fat: 3g
- Fiber: 4g

MIXED GREENS WITH LEMON VINAIGRETTE
(Serves 2 | 5 mins)

INGREDIENTS

- 2 cups mixed salad greens
- 1 tbsp olive oil
- Juice of 1/2 lemon
- Salt and pepper to taste

DIRECTIONS

1. Place greens in a bowl.
2. Mix olive oil, lemon juice, salt, and pepper.
3. Drizzle dressing over greens.
4. Toss gently before serving.

NUTRITIONAL INFO

- Calories: 50
- Carbs: 2g
- Fat: 4g
- Fiber: 1g

ROASTED BUTTERNUT SQUASH WITH THYME

(Serves 2 | 25 mins)

INGREDIENTS

- 1 cup butternut squash (cubed)
- 1 tbsp olive oil
- 1 tsp dried thyme
- Salt and pepper to taste

DIRECTIONS

1. Preheat oven to 400°F (200°C).
2. Toss squash with olive oil, thyme, salt, and pepper.
3. Spread on a baking sheet.
4. Roast for 20-25 mins until tender.
5. Serve warm.

NUTRITIONAL INFO

- Calories: 70
- Carbs: 12g
- Fat: 3g
- Fiber: 2g

ROASTED SWEET POTATO AND SPINACH SALAD

(Serves 2 | 20 mins)

INGREDIENTS

- 1 medium sweet potato (cubed)
- 1 tbsp olive oil
- 2 cups baby spinach
- 1 tbsp sunflower seeds
- Salt and pepper to taste

DIRECTIONS

1. Preheat oven to 400°F (200°C).
2. Toss sweet potato cubes with olive oil, salt, and pepper.
3. Roast for 15-20 mins until tender.
4. Mix roasted sweet potatoes with spinach and sunflower seeds.
5. Serve warm or cold.

NUTRITIONAL INFO

- Calories: 150
- Carbs: 25g
- Fat: 6g
- Fiber: 4g

STEAMED BROCCOLI WITH LEMON OLIVE OIL

(Serves 2 | 20 mins)

INGREDIENTS

- 2 cups broccoli florets
- 1 tbsp olive oil
- Juice of 1/2 lemon
- Salt to taste

DIRECTIONS

1. Steam broccoli for 4-5 mins until tender.
2. Mix olive oil, lemon juice, and salt.
3. Drizzle dressing over steamed broccoli.
4. Serve warm.

NUTRITIONAL INFO

- Calories: 70
- Carbs: 7g
- Fat: 4g
- Fiber: 3g

CABBAGE AND CARROT SLAW

(Serves 2 | 5 mins)

INGREDIENTS

- 1 cup cabbage (shredded)
- 1 carrot (grated)
- 1 tbsp apple cider vinegar
- 1 tbsp olive oil
- Salt and pepper to taste

DIRECTIONS

1. Combine cabbage and carrot in a bowl.
2. Mix vinegar, olive oil, salt, and pepper.
3. Pour dressing over veggies.
4. Toss well and serve immediately.

NUTRITIONAL INFO

- Calories: 50
- Carbs: 6g
- Fat: 4g
- Fiber: 2g

ZUCCHINI NOODLES WITH CHERRY TOMATOES

(Serves 2 | 10 mins)

INGREDIENTS

- 1 zucchini (spiralized into noodles)
- 1/2 cup cherry tomatoes (halved)
- 1 tbsp olive oil
- Fresh basil leaves (chopped)
- Salt and pepper to taste

DIRECTIONS

1. Heat olive oil in a pan over medium heat.
2. Add zucchini noodles and sauté for 2 mins.
3. Add cherry tomatoes and cook for 1-2 mins more.
4. Season with salt, pepper, and fresh basil before serving.

NUTRITIONAL INFO

- Calories: 60
- Carbs: 5g
- Fat: 4g
- Fiber: 2g

ROASTED PUMPKIN WITH ROSEMARY

(Serves 2 | 20 mins)

INGREDIENTS

- 1 cup pumpkin (cubed)
- 1 tbsp olive oil
- 1 tsp dried rosemary
- Salt and pepper to taste

DIRECTIONS

1. Preheat oven to 400°F (200°C).
2. Toss pumpkin cubes with olive oil, rosemary, salt, and pepper.
3. Spread on a baking sheet and roast for 15-20 mins.
4. Serve warm as a side dish.

NUTRITIONAL INFO

- Calories: 80
- Carbs: 10g
- Fat: 4g
- Fiber: 3g

GREEN BEAN AND ALMOND SALAD

(Serves 2 | 10 mins)

INGREDIENTS

- 2 cups green beans (trimmed)
- 2 tbsp sliced almonds
- 1 tbsp olive oil
- Salt and pepper to taste

DIRECTIONS

1. Steam green beans until tender (5-6 mins).
2. Mix green beans with olive oil, salt, and pepper.
3. Top with sliced almonds.
4. Serve warm or chilled.

NUTRITIONAL INFO

- Calories: 90
- Carbs: 6g
- Fat: 7g
- Fiber: 3g

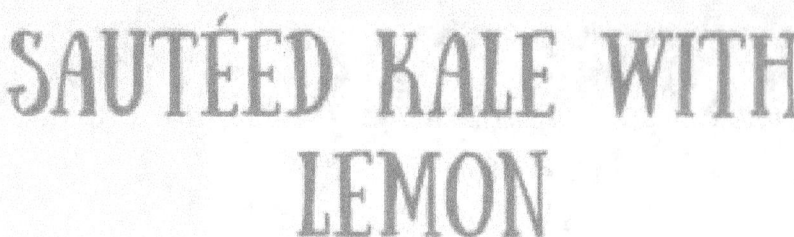

SAUTÉED KALE WITH LEMON

(Serves 2 | 10 mins)

INGREDIENTS

- 2 cups kale (chopped)
- 1 tbsp olive oil
- Juice of 1/2 lemon
- Salt and pepper to taste

DIRECTIONS

1. Heat olive oil in a pan over medium heat.
2. Add kale and sauté until wilted (3-4 mins).
3. Season with salt, pepper, and lemon juice.
4. Serve warm.

NUTRITIONAL INFO

- Calories: 60
- Carbs: 5g
- Fat: 4g
- Fiber: 2g

CARROT AND CUCUMBER RIBBONS SALAD

(Serves 2 | 5 mins)

INGREDIENTS

- 2 carrots (peeled into ribbons)
- 1 cucumber (peeled into ribbons)
- 1 tbsp rice vinegar
- 1 tbsp olive oil
- Salt to taste

DIRECTIONS

1. Combine carrot and cucumber ribbons in a bowl.
2. Mix rice vinegar, olive oil, and salt.
3. Drizzle dressing over ribbons.
4. Toss gently and serve immediately.

NUTRITIONAL INFO

- Calories: 50
- Carbs: 5g
- Fat: 4g
- Fiber: 1g

GRILLED BELL PEPPER SALAD

(Serves 2 | 15 mins)

INGREDIENTS

- 1 red bell pepper (quartered)
- 1 yellow bell pepper (quartered)
- 1 tbsp olive oil
- Fresh parsley (chopped)
- Salt and pepper to taste

DIRECTIONS

1. Brush bell peppers with olive oil, salt, and pepper.
2. Grill on medium heat until charred (3-4 mins per side).
3. Slice grilled peppers and mix with parsley.
4. Serve warm or cold.

NUTRITIONAL INFO

- Calories: 70
- Carbs: 8g
- Fat: 4g
- Fiber: 2g

ROASTED FENNEL WITH THYME

(Serves 2 | 20 mins)

INGREDIENTS

- 1 fennel bulb (sliced)
- 1 tbsp olive oil
- 1 tsp dried thyme
- Salt and pepper to taste

DIRECTIONS

1. Preheat oven to 400°F (200°C).
2. Toss fennel slices with olive oil, thyme, salt, and pepper.
3. Roast on a baking sheet for 15-20 mins until tender.
4. Serve as a side dish.

NUTRITIONAL INFO

- Calories: 50
- Carbs: 7g
- Fat: 4g
- Fiber: 2g

ARUGULA AND LEMON SALAD

(Serves 2 | 5 mins)

INGREDIENTS

- 2 cups arugula
- 1 tbsp olive oil
- Juice of 1/2 lemon
- Salt and pepper to taste

DIRECTIONS

1. Place arugula in a bowl.
2. Mix olive oil, lemon juice, salt, and pepper.
3. Drizzle dressing over arugula.
4. Toss and serve immediately.

NUTRITIONAL INFO

- Calories: 40
- Carbs: 2g
- Fat: 4g
- Fiber: 1g

Snacks And Dessert Recipes

CHOCOLATE-DIPPED STRAWBERRIES

(Serves 2 | 10 mins)

INGREDIENTS

- 1/2 cup dark chocolate chips (Low FODMAP)
- 10 strawberries (washed and dried)
- 1 tsp coconut oil

DIRECTIONS

1. Melt chocolate chips and coconut oil in a microwave-safe bowl.
2. Stir until smooth.
3. Dip strawberries in melted chocolate.
4. Place on a parchment-lined tray.
5. Chill in the refrigerator for 10 mins until set.

NUTRITIONAL INFO

- Calories: 100
- Carbs: 15g
- Fat: 5g
- Fiber: 3g

CINNAMON ALMONDS

(Serves 2 | 10 mins)

INGREDIENTS

- 1 cup almonds
- 1 tbsp maple syrup
- 1 tsp ground cinnamon
- Pinch of salt

DIRECTIONS

1. Preheat oven to 350°F (175°C).
2. Toss almonds with maple syrup, cinnamon, and salt.
3. Spread on a baking sheet.
4. Bake for 8-10 mins until toasted.
5. Let cool before serving.

NUTRITIONAL INFO

- Calories: 180
- Carbs: 7g
- Fat: 15g
- Protein: 6g

PEANUT BUTTER BANANA BITES

(Serves 1 | 5 mins)

INGREDIENTS

- 1 ripe banana (sliced)
- 2 tbsp natural peanut butter
- 1 tbsp unsweetened coconut flakes

DIRECTIONS

1. Spread peanut butter on banana slices.
2. Sandwich two slices together.
3. Roll in coconut flakes.
4. Chill for a firmer texture if desired.

NUTRITIONAL INFO

- Calories: 150
- Carbs: 20g
- Fat: 7g
- Fiber: 3g

COCONUT MACAROONS

(Serves 3 | 20 mins)

INGREDIENTS

- 1 cup unsweetened shredded coconut
- 2 egg whites
- 2 tbsp maple syrup
- 1/2 tsp vanilla extract

DIRECTIONS

1. Preheat oven to 350°F (175°C).
2. Mix all ingredients in a bowl until combined.
3. Form small balls and place on a lined baking sheet.
4. Bake for 15-20 mins until golden.
5. Cool before serving.

NUTRITIONAL INFO

- Calories: 100
- Carbs: 6g
- Fat: 8g
- Protein: 2g

BAKED APPLE SLICES

(Serves 2 | 15 mins)

INGREDIENTS

- 1 apple (cored and sliced)
- 1 tbsp maple syrup
- 1/2 tsp cinnamon
- 1 tsp coconut oil

DIRECTIONS

1. Preheat oven to 375°F (190°C).
2. Toss apple slices with maple syrup, cinnamon, and coconut oil.
3. Spread on a baking sheet.
4. Bake for 10-15 mins until soft.
5. Serve warm or chilled.

NUTRITIONAL INFO

- Calories: 80
- Carbs: 15g
- Fat: 3g
- Fiber: 2g

BLUEBERRY YOGURT PARFAIT

(Serves 1 | 5 mins)

INGREDIENTS

- 1/2 cup lactose-free yogurt
- 1/4 cup blueberries
- 1 tbsp gluten-free granola
- 1 tsp maple syrup

DIRECTIONS

1. Layer yogurt, blueberries, and granola in a cup.
2. Drizzle with maple syrup.
3. Serve immediately or chill.

NUTRITIONAL INFO

- Calories: 120
- Carbs: 18g
- Fat: 4g
- Protein: 4g

RICE CAKE WITH AVOCADO AND SEA SALT

(Serves 1 | 5 mins)

INGREDIENTS

- 1 plain rice cake
- 1/2 ripe avocado
- Pinch of sea salt
- Squeeze of lemon juice

DIRECTIONS

1. Mash avocado and mix with lemon juice.
2. Spread avocado on rice cake.
3. Sprinkle with sea salt.
4. Serve immediately.

NUTRITIONAL INFO

- Calories: 90
- Carbs: 12g
- Fat: 5g
- Fiber: 3g

CARROT STICKS WITH HUMMUS

(Serves 1 | 5 mins)

INGREDIENTS

- 1 carrot (peeled and cut into sticks)
- 2 tbsp Low FODMAP hummus (without garlic)
- 1 tsp olive oil (for drizzling, optional)

DIRECTIONS

1. Arrange carrot sticks on a plate.
2. Serve with a side of hummus.
3. Optional: Drizzle hummus with olive oil.

NUTRITIONAL INFO

- Calories: 80
- Carbs: 10g
- Fat: 4g
- Fiber: 3g

KIWI AND COCONUT POPSICLES

(Serves 3 | 5 mins prep + 3 hrs freezing)

INGREDIENTS

- 2 ripe kiwis (peeled and sliced)
- 1 cup coconut milk (canned, low-fat)
- 1 tbsp maple syrup

DIRECTIONS

1. Blend kiwi, coconut milk, and maple syrup until smooth.
2. Pour mixture into popsicle molds.
3. Freeze for at least 3 hours until set.
4. Remove from molds and serve.

NUTRITIONAL INFO

- Calories: 60
- Carbs: 8g
- Fat: 3g
- Fiber: 1g

ORANGE DARK CHOCOLATE BARK

(Serves 2 | 10 mins prep + 20 mins chilling)

INGREDIENTS

- 1/2 cup dark chocolate chips (Low FODMAP)
- Zest of 1 orange
- 1 tbsp chopped almonds

DIRECTIONS

1. Melt chocolate chips in a microwave-safe bowl.
2. Stir in orange zest.
3. Spread chocolate on a parchment-lined tray.
4. Sprinkle with almonds.
5. Chill for 20 mins until set, then break into pieces.

NUTRITIONAL INFO

- Calories: 100
- Carbs: 10g
- Fat: 6g
- Fiber: 2g

BAKED BANANA CHIPS

(Serves 2 | 30 mins)

INGREDIENTS

- 2 ripe bananas (sliced thinly)
- 1 tbsp lemon juice
- 1 tsp coconut oil (melted)

DIRECTIONS

1. Preheat oven to 250°F (120°C).
2. Toss banana slices with lemon juice and coconut oil.
3. Arrange on a parchment-lined baking sheet.
4. Bake for 25-30 mins until crisp.
5. Cool before serving.

NUTRITIONAL INFO

- Calories: 80
- Carbs: 20g
- Fat: 1g
- Fiber: 2g

COCONUT CHIA PUDDING

Serves 2 | 5 mins prep + 4 hrs chilling)

INGREDIENTS

- 1 cup coconut milk (canned, low-fat)
- 2 tbsp chia seeds
- 1 tbsp maple syrup
- 1 tsp vanilla extract

DIRECTIONS

1. Mix coconut milk, chia seeds, maple syrup, and vanilla.
2. Let sit for 5 mins, then stir again to prevent clumping.
3. Cover and refrigerate for at least 4 hrs or overnight.
4. Serve chilled, topped with fresh fruit if desired.

NUTRITIONAL INFO

- Calories: 120
- Carbs: 8g
- Fat: 7g
- Protein: 3g

LACTOSE-FREE YOGURT WITH KIWI AND WALNUTS

(Serves 1 | 5 mins)

INGREDIENTS

- 1/2 cup lactose-free yogurt
- 1 kiwi (sliced)
- 1 tbsp chopped walnuts
- 1 tsp maple syrup (optional)

DIRECTIONS

1. Scoop yogurt into a bowl.
2. Top with kiwi slices and chopped walnuts.
3. Drizzle with maple syrup if desired.
4. Serve immediately.

NUTRITIONAL INFO

- Calories: 140
- Carbs: 10g
- Fat: 7g
- Protein: 5g

BAKED CINNAMON APPLE CHIPS

(Serves 2 | 45 mins)

INGREDIENTS

- 1 apple (cored and thinly sliced)
- 1 tsp ground cinnamon

DIRECTIONS

1. Preheat oven to 225°F (110°C).
2. Arrange apple slices on a baking sheet lined with parchment.
3. Sprinkle with cinnamon.
4. Bake for 40-45 mins, flipping halfway through.
5. Cool and serve.

NUTRITIONAL INFO

- Calories: 50
- Carbs: 12g
- Fat: 0g
- Fiber: 2g

CHOCOLATE AVOCADO MOUSSE

(Serves 2 | 5 mins)

INGREDIENTS

- 1 ripe avocado
- 2 tbsp cocoa powder (unsweetened)
- 2 tbsp maple syrup
- 1/2 tsp vanilla extract

DIRECTIONS

1. Blend avocado, cocoa powder, maple syrup, and vanilla until smooth.
2. Spoon into serving bowls.
3. Chill for 10 mins before serving.

NUTRITIONAL INFO

- Calories: 150
- Carbs: 14g
- Fat: 10g
- Fiber: 4g

MIXED BERRY SMOOTHIE

(Serves 1 | 5 mins)

INGREDIENTS

- 1/2 cup blueberries (fresh or frozen)
- 1/2 cup strawberries (fresh or frozen)
- 1/2 cup lactose-free milk
- 1 tbsp chia seeds

DIRECTIONS

1. Combine all ingredients in a blender.
2. Blend until smooth.
3. Pour into a glass and serve immediately.

NUTRITIONAL INFO

- Calories: 110
- Carbs: 18g
- Fat: 3g
- Protein: 4g

RICE CAKE WITH PEANUT BUTTER AND BLUEBERRIES

(Serves 1 | 5 mins)

INGREDIENTS

- 1 plain rice cake
- 1 tbsp natural peanut butter
- 1/4 cup blueberries

DIRECTIONS

1. Spread peanut butter on the rice cake.
2. Top with blueberries.
3. Serve immediately.

NUTRITIONAL INFO

- Calories: 130
- Carbs: 15g
- Fat: 7g
- Fiber: 3g

FROZEN GRAPE SNACK

(Serves 2 | 5 mins prep + 1 hr freezing)

INGREDIENTS

- 1 cup seedless grapes (washed)
- 1 tsp lemon juice

DIRECTIONS

1. Toss grapes with lemon juice.
2. Spread on a tray lined with parchment.
3. Freeze for 1 hr or until firm.
4. Enjoy as a cool, refreshing snack.

NUTRITIONAL INFO

- Calories: 60
- Carbs: 15g
- Fat: 0g
- Fiber: 1g

ALMOND BUTTER APPLE SLICES

(Serves 1 | 5 mins)

INGREDIENTS

- 1 apple (cored and sliced)
- 1 tbsp almond butter
- 1 tsp cinnamon

DIRECTIONS

1. Arrange apple slices on a plate.
2. Drizzle with almond butter.
3. Sprinkle with cinnamon.
4. Serve immediately.

NUTRITIONAL INFO

- Calories: 110
- Carbs: 18g
- Fat: 5g
- Fiber: 4g

LEMON BLUEBERRY MUFFINS (GLUTEN-FREE)

(Serves 3 | 20 mins)

INGREDIENTS

- 1/2 cup gluten-free flour
- 1/2 tsp baking powder
- 1 egg
- 1/4 cup blueberries
- Zest of 1 lemon

DIRECTIONS

1. Preheat oven to 350°F (175°C).
2. Mix flour, baking powder, egg, and lemon zest.
3. Fold in blueberries.
4. Spoon batter into muffin cups.
5. Bake for 15-18 mins until golden.

NUTRITIONAL INFO

- Calories: 80
- Carbs: 12g
- Fat: 2g
- Protein: 3g

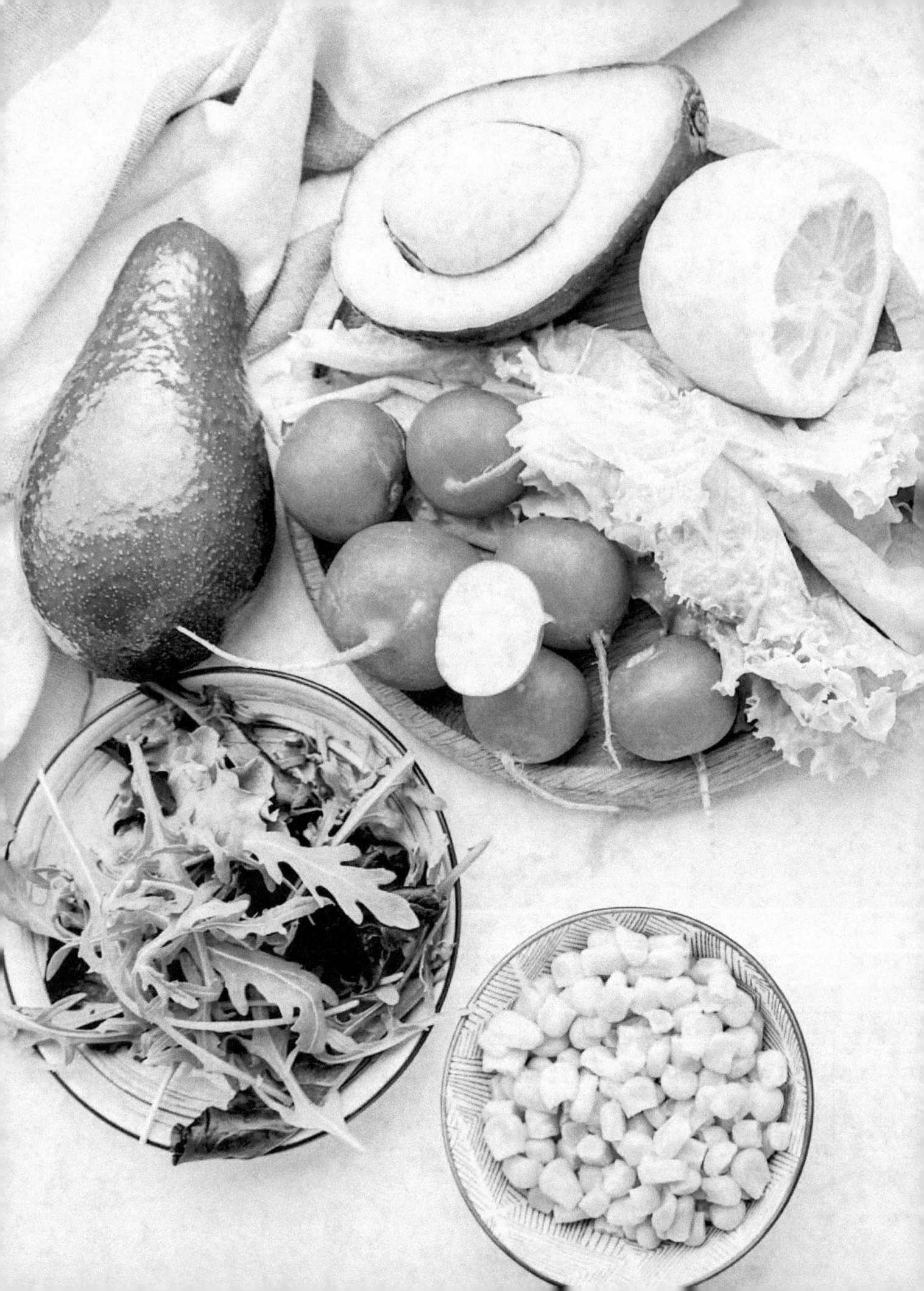

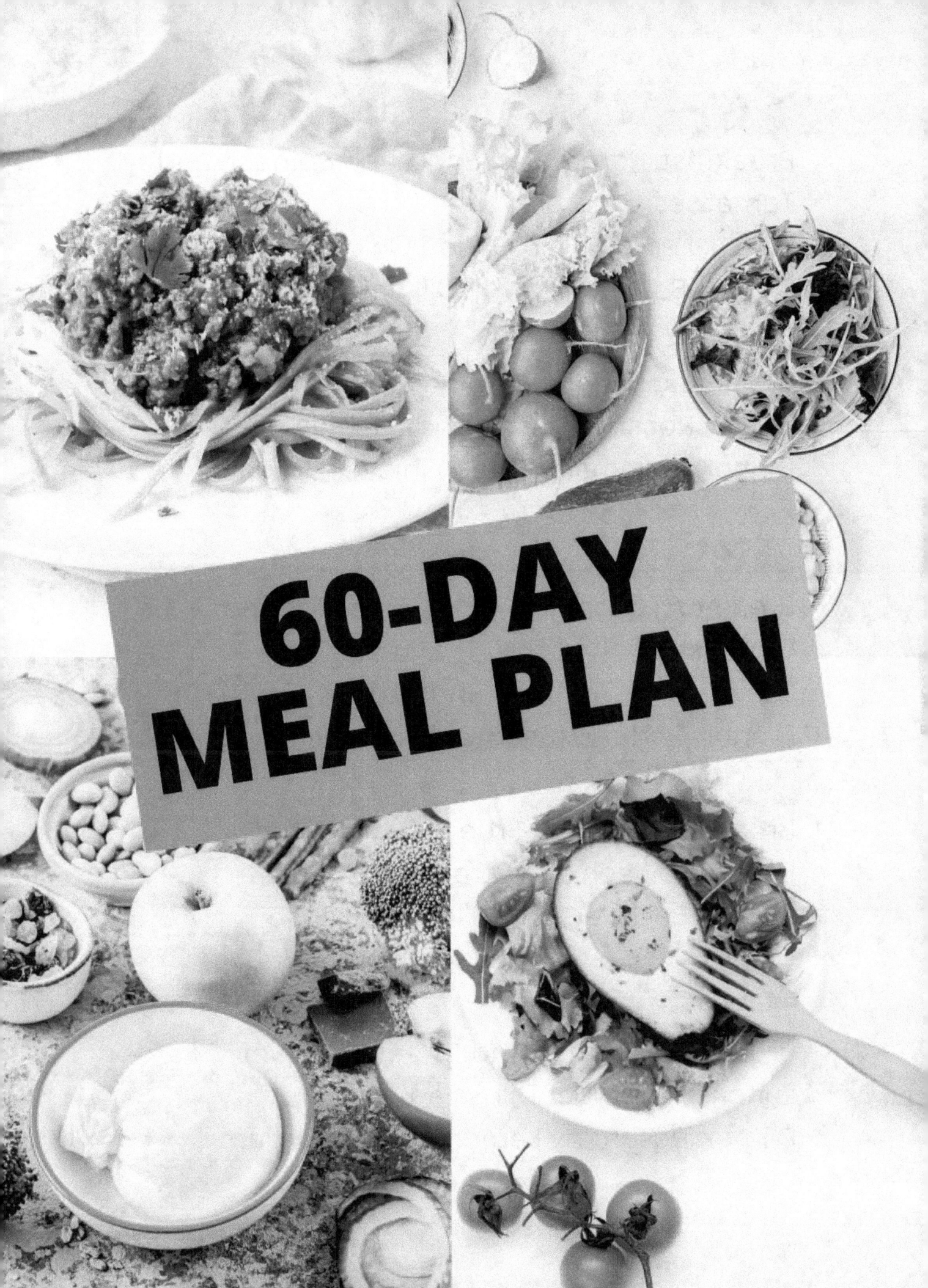

60-DAY MEAL PLAN

Meal Plan

DAY 1

Breakfast: Scrambled Eggs with Spinach and Tomatoes
Lunch: Lemon Herb Grilled Chicken Breast
Dinner: Baked Cod with Dill and Lemon

DAY 2

Breakfast: Banana Almond Smoothie
Lunch: Roasted Carrot and Zucchini Salad
Dinner: Rosemary Baked Chicken Thighs

DAY 3

Breakfast: Oatmeal with Blueberries and Cinnamon
Lunch: Garlic-Infused Shrimp Stir-Fry
Dinner: Garlic-Infused Chicken Stir-Fry

DA 4

Breakfast: Lactose-Free Yogurt Parfait
Lunch: Spinach and Strawberry Salad
Dinner: Basil Lemon Grilled Swordfish

DAY 5

Breakfast: Spinach and Cheese Omelet
Lunch: Cucumber Dill Salad
Dinner: Rosemary Lemon Turkey Burgers

Meal Plan

DAY 6

Breakfast: Peanut Butter Rice Cakes
Lunch: Roasted Bell Peppers and Eggplant
Dinner: Paprika Baked Turkey Breast

DAY 7

Breakfast: Quinoa Breakfast Bowl
Lunch: Simple Tomato and Basil Salad
Dinner: Balsamic Glazed Chicken Drumsticks

DAY 8

Breakfast: Coconut Chia Pudding
Lunch: Roasted Green Beans with Lemon Zest
Dinner: Turmeric Lemon Roasted Chicken Wings

DA 9

Breakfast: Tomato and Basil Frittata
Lunch: Grilled Asparagus with Sea Salt
Dinner: Grilled Jerk-Spiced Chicken Thighs

DAY 10

Breakfast: Pumpkin Spice Overnight Oats
Lunch: Carrot and Parsnip Mash
Dinner: Cumin Spiced Grilled Turkey Breast

DAY 11

Breakfast: Avocado Toast with Poached Egg
Lunch: Mixed Greens with Lemon Vinaigrette
Dinner: Maple Mustard Chicken Breasts

DAY 12

Breakfast: Fruit and Cottage Cheese Bowl
Lunch: Roasted Butternut Squash with Thyme
Dinner: Citrus Grilled Chicken Thighs

DAY 13

Breakfast: Almond Flour Pancakes
Lunch: Roasted Sweet Potato and Spinach Salad
Dinner: Rosemary Lemon Turkey Burgers

DA 14

Breakfast: Quinoa Breakfast Porridge
Lunch: Steamed Broccoli with Lemon Olive Oil
Dinner: Thyme Roasted Chicken Drumsticks

DAY 15

Breakfast: Egg and Bell Pepper Cups
Lunch: Cabbage and Carrot Slaw
Dinner: Basil Pesto Baked Chicken

DAY 16

Breakfast: Buckwheat Porridge with Strawberries
Lunch: Zucchini Noodles with Cherry Tomatoes
Dinner: Honey Lime Grilled Turkey Cutlets

DAY 17

Breakfast: Berry Chia Pudding
Lunch: Roasted Pumpkin with Rosemary
Dinner: Sage Baked Chicken Breasts

DAY 18

Breakfast: Spinach and Feta Breakfast Wrap
Lunch: Green Bean and Almond Salad
Dinner: Teriyaki Turkey Stir-Fry

DA 19

Breakfast: Maple-Cinnamon Rice Porridge
Lunch: Sautéed Kale with Lemon
Dinner: Oregano Lemon Chicken Thighs

DAY 20

Breakfast: Tomato & Basil Breakfast Skillet
Lunch: Carrot and Cucumber Ribbons Salad
Dinner: Cumin Lime Grilled Chicken

DAY 21

Breakfast: Scrambled Eggs with Spinach and Tomatoes
Lunch: Grilled Bell Pepper Salad
Dinner: Cilantro Lime Turkey Meatballs

DAY 22

Breakfast: Banana Almond Smoothie
Lunch: Roasted Fennel with Thyme
Dinner: Garlic-Infused Mackerel with Herbs

DAY 23

Breakfast: Oatmeal with Blueberries and Cinnamon
Lunch: Arugula and Lemon Salad
Dinner: Lemon-Ginger Baked Trout

DA 24

Breakfast: Lactose-Free Yogurt Parfait
Lunch: Mixed Greens with Lemon Vinaigrette
Dinner: Herb-Crusted Baked Haddock

DAY 25

Breakfast: Spinach and Cheese Omelet
Lunch: Roasted Sweet Potato and Spinach Salad
Dinner: Basil Lemon Grilled Swordfish

DAY 26

Breakfast: Peanut Butter Rice Cakes
Lunch: Sautéed Kale with Lemon
Dinner: Crispy Baked Sole Fillets

DAY 27

Breakfast: Quinoa Breakfast Bowl
Lunch: Zucchini Noodles with Cherry Tomatoes
Dinner: Ginger Soy Shrimp Sauté

DAY 28

Breakfast: Coconut Chia Pudding
Lunch: Cabbage and Carrot Slaw
Dinner: Lemon Dill Poached Haddock

DA 29

Breakfast: Tomato and Basil Frittata
Lunch: Grilled Asparagus with Sea Salt
Dinner: Baked Mahi-Mahi with Fresh Herbs

DAY 30

Breakfast: Pumpkin Spice Overnight Oats
Lunch: Roasted Carrot and Zucchini Salad
Dinner: Paprika Grilled Prawns

DAY 31

Breakfast: Avocado Toast with Poached Egg
Lunch: Spinach and Strawberry Salad
Dinner: Sesame-Crusted Salmon

DAY 32

Breakfast: Fruit and Cottage Cheese Bowl
Lunch: Cucumber Dill Salad
Dinner: Lime and Cilantro Grilled Tilapia

DAY 33

Breakfast: Almond Flour Pancakes
Lunch: Roasted Bell Peppers and Eggplant
Dinner: Herb-Roasted Sea Bass

DA 34

Breakfast: Quinoa Breakfast Porridge
Lunch: Mixed Greens with Lemon Vinaigrette
Dinner: Cumin-Spiced Grilled Halibut

DAY 35

Breakfast: Egg and Bell Pepper Cups
Lunch: Roasted Green Beans with Lemon Zest
Dinner: Chili Lime Grilled Tuna

DAY 36

Breakfast: Buckwheat Porridge with Strawberries
Lunch: Grilled Asparagus with Sea Salt
Dinner: Lemon-Ginger Baked Trout

DAY 37

Breakfast: Berry Chia Pudding
Lunch: Arugula and Lemon Salad
Dinner: Sesame-Crusted Tuna Steaks

DAY 38

Breakfast: Spinach and Feta Breakfast Wrap
Lunch: Roasted Butternut Squash with Thyme
Dinner: Baked Tilapia with Paprika and Lemon

DA 39

Breakfast: Maple-Cinnamon Rice Porridge
Lunch: Steamed Broccoli with Lemon Olive Oil
Dinner: Cilantro Lime Shrimp Skewers

DAY 40

Breakfast: Tomato & Basil Breakfast Skillet
Lunch: Roasted Sweet Potato and Spinach Salad
Dinner: Baked Mahi-Mahi with Fresh Herbs

Meal Plan

DAY 41

Breakfast: Scrambled Eggs with Spinach and Tomatoes
Lunch: Cabbage and Carrot Slaw
Dinner: Garlic-Infused Shrimp Stir-Fry

DAY 42

Breakfast: Banana Almond Smoothie
Lunch: Zucchini Noodles with Cherry Tomatoes
Dinner: Baked Cod with Dill and Lemon

DAY 43

Breakfast: Oatmeal with Blueberries and Cinnamon
Lunch: Grilled Bell Pepper Salad
Dinner: Rosemary Baked Chicken Thighs

DA 44

Breakfast: Lactose-Free Yogurt Parfait
Lunch: Roasted Pumpkin with Rosemary
Dinner: Ginger Lime Turkey Meatballs

DAY 45

Breakfast: Spinach and Cheese Omelet
Lunch: Mixed Greens with Lemon Vinaigrette
Dinner: Balsamic Glazed Chicken Drumsticks

Meal Plan

DAY 46
Breakfast: Peanut Butter Rice Cakes
Lunch: Sautéed Kale with Lemon
Dinner: Herb-Crusted Baked Haddock

DAY 47
Breakfast: Quinoa Breakfast Bowl
Lunch: Carrot and Cucumber Ribbons Salad
Dinner: Rosemary Lemon Turkey Burgers

DAY 48
Breakfast: Coconut Chia Pudding
Lunch: Roasted Fennel with Thyme
Dinner: Lemon Dill Poached Haddock

DA 49
Breakfast: Tomato and Basil Frittata
Lunch: Roasted Carrot and Zucchini Salad
Dinner: Basil Lemon Grilled Swordfish

DAY 50
Breakfast: Pumpkin Spice Overnight Oats
Lunch: Cucumber Dill Salad
Dinner: Sesame-Crusted Salmon

DAY 51

Breakfast: Avocado Toast with Poached Egg
Lunch: Roasted Green Beans with Lemon Zest
Dinner: Cumin-Spiced Grilled Halibut

DAY 52

Breakfast: Fruit and Cottage Cheese Bowl
Lunch: Roasted Bell Peppers and Eggplant
Dinner: Lime and Cilantro Grilled Tilapia

DAY 53

Breakfast: Almond Flour Pancakes
Lunch: Mixed Greens with Lemon Vinaigrette
Dinner: Chili Lime Grilled Tuna

DA 54

Breakfast: Quinoa Breakfast Porridge
Lunch: Steamed Broccoli with Lemon Olive Oil
Dinner: Herb-Roasted Sea Bass

DAY 55

Breakfast: Egg and Bell Pepper Cups
Lunch: Arugula and Lemon Salad
Dinner: Teriyaki Turkey Stir-Fry

Meal Plan

DAY 56

Breakfast: Buckwheat Porridge with Strawberries
Lunch: Roasted Sweet Potato and Spinach Salad
Dinner: Maple Mustard Chicken Breasts

DAY 57

Breakfast: Berry Chia Pudding
Lunch: Cabbage and Carrot Slaw
Dinner: Cilantro Lime Shrimp Skewers

DAY 58

Breakfast: Spinach and Feta Breakfast Wrap
Lunch: Grilled Asparagus with Sea Salt
Dinner: Baked Mahi-Mahi with Fresh Herbs

DA 59

Breakfast: Maple-Cinnamon Rice Porridge
Lunch: Roasted Butternut Squash with Thyme
Dinner: Rosemary Lemon Turkey Burgers

DAY 60

Breakfast: Tomato & Basil Breakfast Skillet
Lunch: Zucchini Noodles with Cherry Tomatoes
Dinner: Garlic-Infused Chicken Stir-Fry

LIST OF INGREDIENTS

Below is a comprehensive list of ingredients compiled from all the provided Low FODMAP recipes, organized into categories for easy reference. This compilation assumes standard ingredients based on the recipe names. Please adjust quantities and verify Low FODMAP portions as needed for your specific dietary requirements.

PROTEINS

Animal-Based Proteins:

- Eggs

Chicken:

- Chicken breasts
- Chicken thighs
- Chicken drumsticks
- Chicken wings

Turkey:

- Turkey breast
- Ground turkey
- Turkey meatballs
- Turkey cutlets
- Turkey burgers

Seafood:

- Shrimp
- Cod
- Scallops
- Tuna steaks
- Tilapia
- Mackerel
- Trout
- Haddock
- Swordfish
- Sole fillets
- Salmon
- Sea bass
- Halibut
- Mahi-Mahi
- Prawns

Dairy Proteins:

Cheeses:

- Feta cheese
- Cheddar cheese
- Parmesan cheese
- Cottage cheese (lactose-free)

Yogurt:

- Lactose-free yogurt
- Non-dairy yogurt (optional)

DAIRY AND ALTERNATIVES

Milk Alternatives:
- Almond milk
- Coconut milk

Butter and Spreads:
- Butter (lactose-free)
- Lactose-free butter
- Peanut butter (natural, no high FODMAP ingredients)
- Almond butter

Other Dairy Products:
- Lactose-free cottage cheese
- Lactose-free yogurt

GRAINS AND ALTERNATIVES

Whole Grains:
- Oats (rolled or steel-cut)
- Quinoa
- Buckwheat groats
- Rice (white or brown)

Gluten-Free Products:
- Gluten-free bread
- Gluten-free tortillas or wraps
- Gluten-free granola
- Gluten-free breadcrumbs
- Gluten-free flour (e.g., almond flour, rice flour)

Rice Products:
- Rice cakes
- Rice flour

NUTS AND SEEDS

Nuts:
- Almonds
- Walnuts
- Pine nuts

Nut Butters:
- Peanut butter
- Almond butter

Seeds:
- Chia seeds
- Sesame seeds

VEGETABLES

Leafy Greens:
- Spinach
- Kale
- Mixed greens (lettuce, arugula, etc.)

Cruciferous and Others:
- Broccoli
- Cabbage
- Fennel bulbs

Root Vegetables:
- Carrots
- Parsnips
- Sweet potatoes
- Butternut squash
- Pumpkin

Alliums (Low FODMAP Alternatives):
- Garlic-infused oil (for flavor without actual garlic)
- Green onions (green parts only)

Other Vegetables:
- Tomatoes
- Bell peppers
- Zucchini
- Cucumbers
- Eggplant
- Green beans
- Asparagus
- Celery (if used, verify portion size)
- Cherry tomatoes

OILS AND FATS

Cooking Oils:
- Olive oil
- Sesame oil
- Coconut oil
- Garlic-infused oil

Vinegars:
- Balsamic vinegar
- Apple cider vinegar
- Rice vinegar

Other Fats:
- Butter (lactose-free)
- Lactose-free butter

SPICES AND HERBS

Herbs:
- **Fresh dill**
- **Fresh basil**
- **Fresh cilantro**
- **Fresh thyme**
- **Rosemary**
- **Oregano**
- **Sage**

Spices:
- **Salt**
- **Black pepper**
- **Cinnamon**
- **Paprika**
- **Ground cumin**
- **Chili powder**
- **Turmeric**
- **Pumpkin spice**

Flavor Enhancers:
- **Fresh ginger**
- **Vanilla extract**
- **Lemon zest**
- **Lime zest**

FRUITS

Berries:
- **Blueberries**
- **Strawberries**
- **Mixed berries**

Citrus Fruits:
- **Lemons**
- **Limes**
- **Oranges**

Other Fruits:
- **Bananas (ensure Low FODMAP portion)**
- **Kiwis**
- **Apples (ensure Low FODMAP portion)**
- **Grapes**
- **Avocado (ensure Low FODMAP portion)**

Dried Fruits:
- **(Use sparingly and verify Low FODMAP compliance)**

MISCELLANEOUS

Baking Essentials:

- Baking powder (gluten-free)
- Baking soda
- Condiments and Sauces:
- Soy sauce or tamari (gluten-free)
- Teriyaki sauce (Low FODMAP, tamari-based)

Others:

- Skewers (for grilling)
- Rice vinegar
- Gelatin (optional for popsicles)
- Low FODMAP broth or white wine (for poaching)

Optional Add-Ins:

- Fresh herbs for garnishing
- Lemon or lime wedges for serving

SWEETENERS

Natural Sweeteners:

- Maple syrup
- Honey (use sparingly and verify Low FODMAP portion)
- Agave nectar

Sugar Alternatives:

- Dark chocolate (ensure Low FODMAP portions)
- Cocoa powder

NOTES AND TIPS

- **Portion Control:** Even Low FODMAP ingredients can become high FODMAP if consumed in large quantities. Always adhere to recommended portion sizes.

- **Substitutions:** Where applicable, use gluten-free or Low FODMAP alternatives to standard ingredients (e.g., gluten-free bread, Low FODMAP hummus).

- **Fresh vs. Dried Herbs:** Fresh herbs are generally preferred for flavor without adding FODMAPs, but dried herbs can be used in smaller quantities.

- **Sweeteners:** Opt for pure maple syrup or other Low FODMAP-approved sweeteners instead of high-fructose options.

- **Cooking Techniques:** Utilize methods like grilling, baking, and steaming to retain the nutritional value of ingredients without adding extra FODMAPs.

- **Check Labels:** Always check product labels to ensure there are no hidden high FODMAP ingredients, especially in processed items like sauces and dressings.

- **Customization:** Feel free to customize the ingredient list based on personal preferences, ensuring all substitutions remain Low FODMAP.

This categorized ingredient list should serve as a helpful reference for meal planning and grocery shopping for your 60-day Low FODMAP diet. Always consult with a healthcare professional or a registered dietitian when making significant changes to your diet.

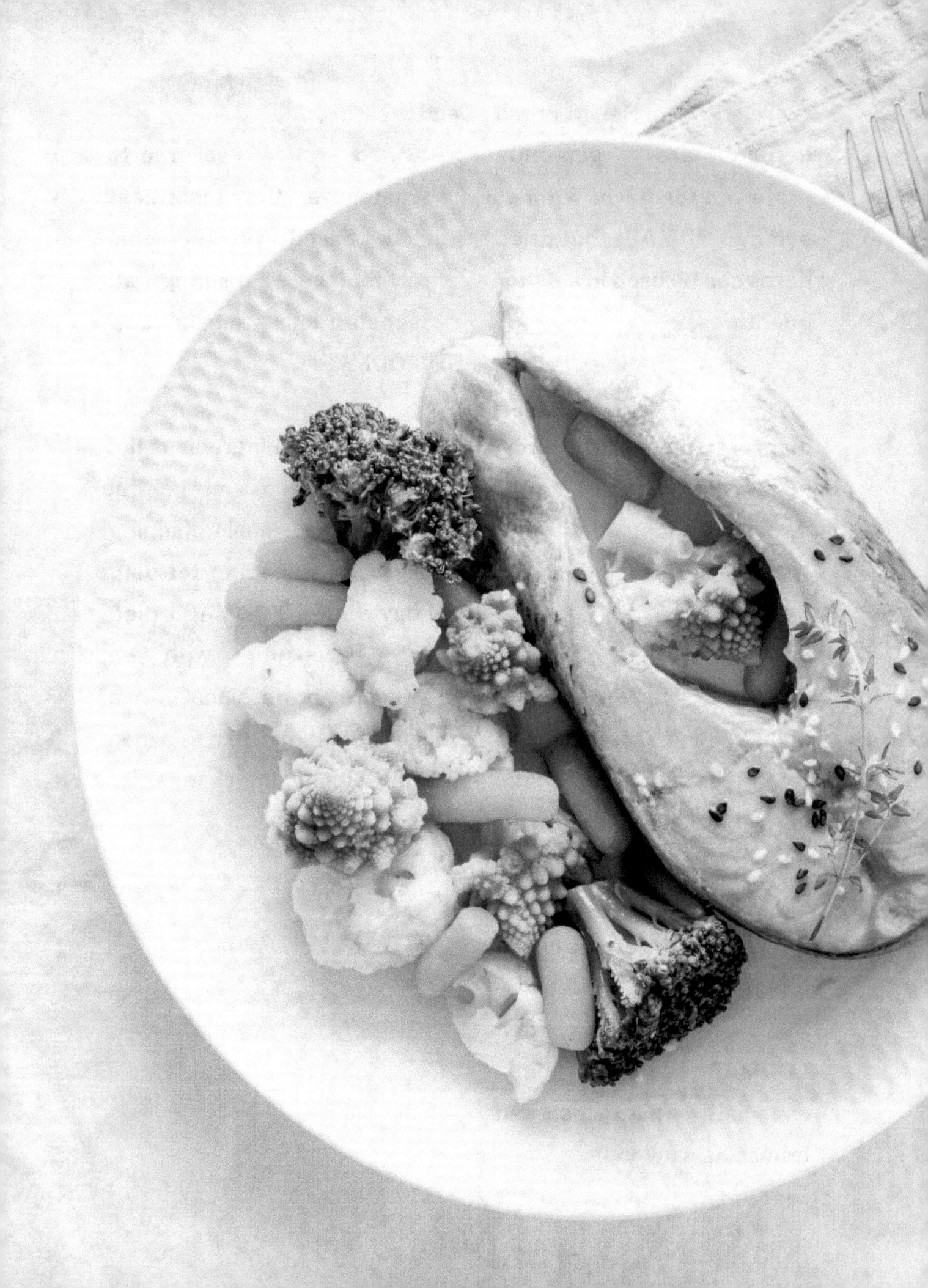

Conclusion

The journey to better digestive health starts with understanding and empowerment, and The Complete Low FODMAP Diet for Beginners is designed to give you both. Throughout this book, you've learned the fundamentals of the Low FODMAP diet, from how FODMAPs affect your gut to the practical steps of elimination, reintroduction, and maintenance. You've explored a variety of delicious and easy-to-make recipes that will nourish your body, ease your symptoms, and allow you to enjoy food again without fear or discomfort.

Embracing the Low FODMAP diet can be a game-changer for your overall well-being. By identifying your trigger foods and building a personalized eating plan, you are giving yourself the opportunity to live a life free from digestive distress. This cookbook is more than a collection of recipes—it's a toolkit for sustainable health, offering meal plans, actionable tips, and the knowledge you need to make informed dietary choices every day.

Remember that adapting to the Low FODMAP lifestyle is a journey, not a quick fix. It requires patience, self-awareness, and a willingness to experiment with new ingredients and flavors. But the reward is worth it: greater control over your gut health, more energy, and a renewed sense of confidence around food.

Motivation is key to your success, so remember this: every step you take on this path is a step toward feeling better, living more freely, and truly enjoying the foods you eat. Empower yourself to make changes today, and embrace the Low FODMAP diet as a positive, lasting shift towards a healthier and happier life. You've got this!

WEEKLY MEAL Planner

DATE

	BREAKFAST	LUNCH	DINNER	SNACKS
MONDAY				
TUESDAY				
WEDNESDAY				
THURSDAY				
FRIDAY				
SATURDAY				
SUNDAY				

WEEKLY MEAL *Planner*

DATE

	BREAKFAST	LUNCH	DINNER	SNACKS
MONDAY				
TUESDAY				
WEDNESDAY				
THURSDAY				
FRIDAY				
SATURDAY				
SUNDAY				

WEEKLY MEAL *Planner*

DATE

	BREAKFAST	LUNCH	DINNER	SNACKS
MONDAY				
TUESDAY				
WEDNESDAY				
THURSDAY				
FRIDAY				
SATURDAY				
SUNDAY				

WEEKLY MEAL Planner

DATE

	BREAKFAST	LUNCH	DINNER	SNACKS
MONDAY				
TUESDAY				
WEDNESDAY				
THURSDAY				
FRIDAY				
SATURDAY				
SUNDAY				

WEEKLY MEAL *Planner*

DATE

	BREAKFAST	LUNCH	DINNER	SNACKS
MONDAY				
TUESDAY				
WEDNESDAY				
THURSDAY				
FRIDAY				
SATURDAY				
SUNDAY				

WEEKLY MEAL *Planner*

DATE

	BREAKFAST	LUNCH	DINNER	SNACKS
MONDAY				
TUESDAY				
WEDNESDAY				
THURSDAY				
FRIDAY				
SATURDAY				
SUNDAY				

WEEKLY MEAL Planner

DATE

	BREAKFAST	LUNCH	DINNER	SNACKS
MONDAY				
TUESDAY				
WEDNESDAY				
THURSDAY				
FRIDAY				
SATURDAY				
SUNDAY				

WEEKLY MEAL *Planner*

DATE

	BREAKFAST	LUNCH	DINNER	SNACKS
MONDAY				
TUESDAY				
WEDNESDAY				
THURSDAY				
FRIDAY				
SATURDAY				
SUNDAY				

WEEKLY MEAL Planner

DATE

	BREAKFAST	LUNCH	DINNER	SNACKS
MONDAY				
TUESDAY				
WEDNESDAY				
THURSDAY				
FRIDAY				
SATURDAY				
SUNDAY				

WEEKLY MEAL *Planner*

DATE

	BREAKFAST	LUNCH	DINNER	SNACKS
MONDAY				
TUESDAY				
WEDNESDAY				
THURSDAY				
FRIDAY				
SATURDAY				
SUNDAY				

THANK YOU FOR READING!

THANK YOU FOR PURCHASING THE COMPLETE LOW FODMAP DIET FOR BEGINNERS
I HOPE YOU FIND THE RECIPES BOTH ENJOYABLE AND HELPFUL ON YOUR CULINARY JOURNEY. YOUR FEEDBACK MEANS A LOT TO ME—PLEASE CONSIDER LEAVING AN HONEST REVIEW TO HELP OTHERS DISCOVER THE BOOK.

WARM REGARDS,

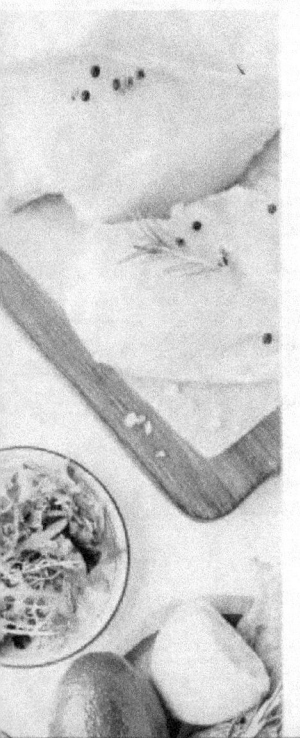
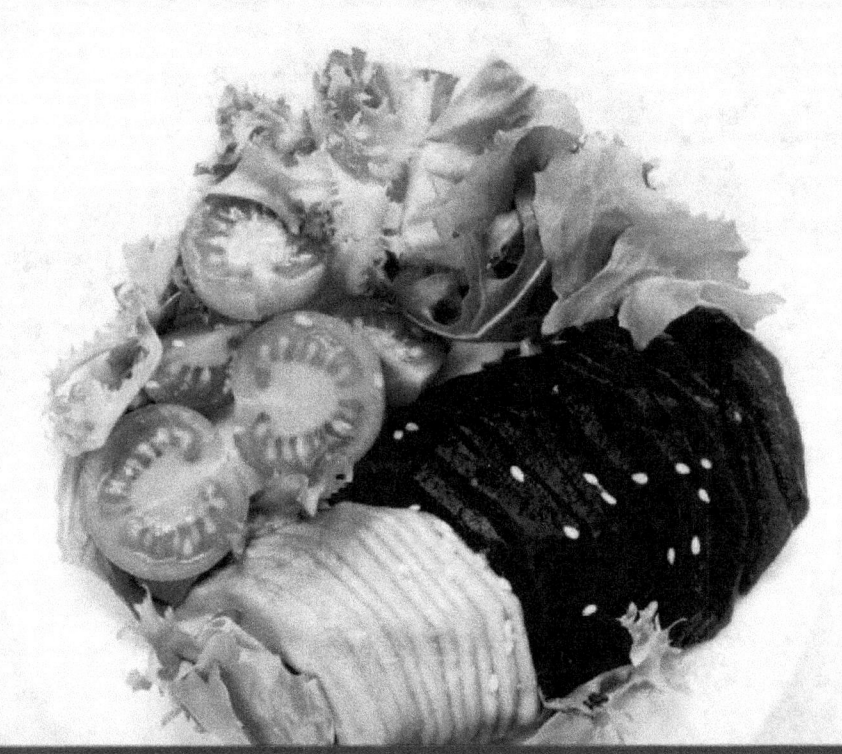
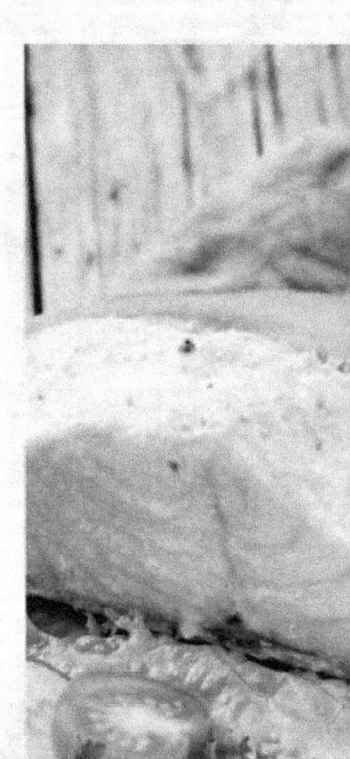

AMADA L. HEATH

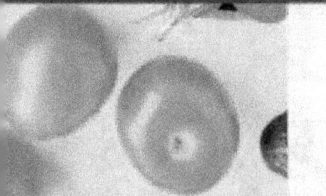

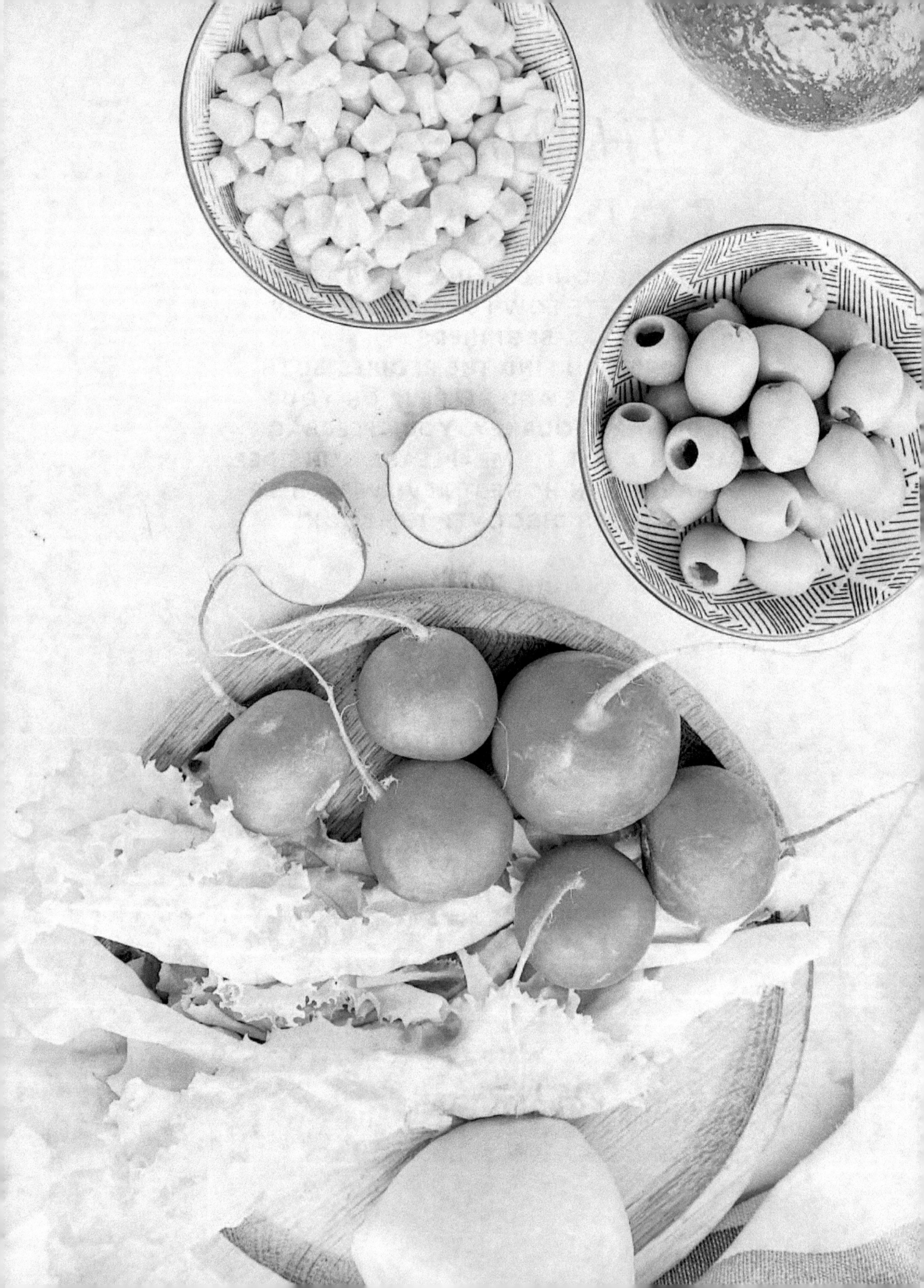

www.ingramcontent.com/pod-product-compliance
Lightning Source LLC
Chambersburg PA
CBHW060414220526
45465CB00008B/2879